Mitral Valve Disease

Editor

TAKESHI KITAI

CARDIOLOGY CLINICS

www.cardiology.theclinics.com

May 2021 • Volume 39 • Number 2

ELSEVIER

1600 John F. Kennedy Boulevard • Suite 1800 • Philadelphia, Pennsylvania, 19103-2899

http://www.theclinics.com

CARDIOLOGY CLINICS Volume 39, Number 2
May 2021 ISSN 0733-8651, ISBN-13: 978-0-323-84918-0

Editor: Joanna Collett
Developmental Editor: Karen Justine Solomon

Cardiology Clinics (ISSN 0733-8651) is published quarterly by Elsevier Inc., 360 Park Avenue South, New York, NY 10010-1710. Months of issue are February, May, August, and November. Business and Editorial Offices: 1600 John F. Kennedy Blvd., Ste. 1800, Philadelphia, PA 19103-2899. Customer Service Office: 3251 Riverport Lane, Maryland Heights, MO 63043. Periodicals postage paid at New York, NY and additional mailing offices. Subscription prices are $359.00 per year for US individuals, $929.00 per year for US institutions, $100.00 per year for US students and residents, $445.00 per year for Canadian individuals, $962.00 per year for Canadian institutions, $466.00 per year for international individuals, $962.00 per year for international institutions, $100.00 per year for Canadian students/residents and $220.00 per year for international students/residents. To receive student/resident rate, orders must be accompanied by name of affiliated institution, data of term, and the *signature* of program/residency coordinator on institution letterhead. Orders will be billed at individual rate until proof of status is received. Foreign air speed delivery is included in all *Clinics* subscription prices. All prices are subject to change without notice. **POSTMASTER:** Send address changes to *Cardiology Clinics*, Elsevier Health Sciences Division, Subscription Customer Service, 3251 Riverport Lane, Maryland Heights, MO 63043. **Customer Service: 1-800-654-2452 (U.S. and Canada); 314-447-8871 (outside U.S. and Canada). Fax: 314-447-8029. E-mail: journalscustomerservice-usa@elsevier.com (for print support); journalsonlinesupport-usa@elsevier.com (for online support).**

Reprints. For copies of 100 or more, of articles in this publication, please contact the Commercial Reprints Department, Elsevier Inc., 360 Park Avenue South, New York, NY 10010-1710. Tel.: 212-633-3874; Fax: 212-633-3820; E-mail: reprints@elsevier.com.

Cardiology Clinics is also published in Spanish by McGraw-Hill Interamericana Editores S. A., P.O. Box 5-237, 06500, Mexico D. F., Mexico; in Portuguese by Reichmann and Alfonso Editores Rio de Janeiro, Brazil; and in Greek by Dimitrios P. Lagos, 8 Pondon Street, GR115-28 Ilissia, Greece.

Cardiology Clinics is covered in *MEDLINE/PubMed (Index Medicus)*, *Excerpta Medica*, *The Cumulative Index to Nursing and Allied Health Literature* (CINAHL).

Contributors

MARC GILLINOV, MD
Department of Thoracic and Cardiovascular Surgery, Cleveland Clinic, Cleveland, Ohio, USA

FRANCESCO GUCCIONE, MD, PhD
Department of Cardiovascular Surgery, GVM Care and Research, Maria Eleonora Hospital, Palermo, Italy

SAMIR R. KAPADIA, MD
Department of Cardiovascular Medicine, Cleveland Clinic Foundation, Cleveland, Ohio, USA

DAE-HEE KIM, MD, PhD
Associate Professor of Medicine, Division of Cardiology, Asan Medical Center, College of Medicine, University of Ulsan, Seoul, Korea

TAKESHI KITAI, MD, PhD, FHFSA
Director of Cardiovascular Care Unit, Department of Cardiovascular Medicine, Kobe City Medical Center General Hospital, Kobe, Japan

TAKASHI KOHNO, MD, PhD
Department of Cardiovascular Medicine, Kyorin University School of Medicine, Tokyo, Japan

SHUN KOHSAKA, MD
Department of Cardiology, Keio University School of Medicine, Tokyo, Japan

TOSHIKO KONDA, BSc
Department of Clinical Technology, Kobe City Medical Center General Hospital, Kobe, Japan

TADAAKI KOYAMA, MD, PhD
Department of Cardiovascular Surgery, Kobe City Medical Center General Hospital, Kobe, Japan

AMAR KRISHNASWAMY, MD
Section Head, Interventional Cardiology, Director, Sones Cardiac Catheterization Laboratories, Program Director, Interventional Cardiology Fellowship, Department of Cardiovascular Medicine, Cleveland Clinic Foundation, Cleveland, Ohio, USA

AKIKO MASUMOTO, MD
Department of Cardiovascular Medicine, Kobe City Medical Center General Hospital, Kobe, Japan

KEISUKE MATSUO, MD
Department of Cardiology, Saitama Medical University, International Medical Center, Saitama, Japan

RHONDA MIYASAKA, MD
Department of Cardiovascular Medicine, Heart and Vascular Institute, Cleveland Clinic, Cleveland, Ohio, USA

VINAYAK NAGARAJA, MBBS, MS, MMed (Clin Epi), FRACP
Department of Cardiovascular Medicine, Cleveland Clinic Foundation, Cleveland, Ohio, USA

YUJI NAGATOMO, MD, PhD
Department of Cardiology, National Defense Medical College, Saitama, Japan

TAKEO NAKAI, MD
Heart Valve Center, Midori Hospital, Kobe, Japan

SHINTARO NAKANO, MD, PhD
Department of Cardiology, Saitama Medical University, International Medical Center, Saitama, Japan

TAIJI OKADA, MD, PhD
Department of Cardiovascular Medicine, Kobe City Medical Center General Hospital, Kobe, Japan

YUKIKATSU OKADA, MD, PhD
Heart Valve Center, Midori Hospital, Kobe, Japan

MITSUHIKO OTA, MD
Department of Cardiovascular Center, Toranomon Hospital, Tokyo, Japan

JAY RAMCHAND, MBBS, BMedSci
Department of Cardiovascular Medicine, Heart and Vascular Institute, Cleveland Clinic, Cleveland, Ohio, USA

MIKE SAJI, MD, PhD
Department of Cardiology, Sakakibara Heart Institute, Tokyo, Japan

TOSHIHIKO SHIBATA, MD, PhD
Department of Cardiovascular Surgery, Osaka City University, Osaka, Japan

SATOSHI SHOJI, MD, PhD
Department of Cardiology, Keio University
School of Medicine, Tokyo, Japan

YOSUKE TAKAHASHI, MD, PhD
Department of Cardiovascular Surgery, Osaka
City University, Osaka, Japan

TOMOKO TANI, MD
Basic Medical Science, Kobe City College of
Nursing, Kobe, Japan

PER WIERUP, MD, PhD
Department of Thoracic and Cardiovascular
Surgery, Cleveland Clinic, Cleveland, Ohio,
USA

Contributors

SATOSHI SHIOIE, MD, PhD
Department of Cardiology, Keio University School of Medicine, Tokyo, Japan

YOSUKE TAKAHASHI, MD, PhD
Department of Cardiovascular Surgery, Osaka City University, Osaka, Japan

TOMOKO TANI, MD
Basel Medical Science, Kobe City College of Nursing, Kobe, Japan

PER WIERUP, MD, PhD
Department of Thoracic and Cardiovascular Surgery, Cleveland Clinic, Cleveland, Ohio, USA

Contents

> Degenerative mitral valve disease represents the most common cause of mitral regurgitation in industrialized countries. When left untreated, patients with severe degenerative mitral regurgitation show a poor clinical outcome. Conversely, a timely and appropriate correction provides a restored life expectancy and a good quality of life. Therefore, in this scenario, surgical mitral valve repair represents the gold standard of treatment. This review aims to analyze the indications, timing, and contemporary surgical techniques of mitral valve repair for degenerative mitral regurgitation. Moreover, the value of heart team approach and centers of excellence for mitral valve repair are also deeply discussed.

> Patient selection is mandatory to successful mitral valve repair in functional mitral valve regurgitation. Preoperative echo evaluation is critical to better evaluate the anatomic modification of the mitral apparatus. In light of recent randomized trials, several patients could benefit from transcatheter mitral therapy. Mitral annuloplasty is not effective in all patients with functional mitral valve regurgitation; meanwhile, adding surgical techniques should be performed to improve the repair durability.

 Video content accompanies this article at http://www.cardiology.theclinics.com.

> The 2 primary objectives of surgery in mitral valve infective endocarditis (IE) are total removal of the infected tissue and reconstruction of cardiac morphology, including repair or replacement of the affected valve. Single-institution series have suggested the feasibility and effectiveness of mitral valve repair (MVrep) over replacement in mitral IE in terms of in-hospital mortality and long-term event-free survival. This article reviews the history, details of the relevant repair techniques, and clinical results of MVrep for mitral IE.

> Infective endocarditis (IE) is a rare but serious condition with a dismal prognosis. One of the keys to improving outcomes is the prompt identification of high-risk patients who have intracardiac and extracardiac (systemic and neurologic) complications. However, as cardiac and extracardiac complications indicating surgery add to the

surgical risk for active IE, controversies surround the optimal indication and timing for surgery, especially in patients presenting neurologic complications. This article reviews the necessary evaluation for patients with suspected IE and proposes a state-of-the-art patient flow chart for evaluation of suspected IE.

In most patients, minimally invasive approaches to mitral valve surgery are technically possible. However, in practice, patient selection is critical to mitigate safety concerns when performing the procedure. In this article, we describe our approach to preoperative assessment for minimally invasive mitral valve surgery candidacy, as well as discussing the technical aspects of procedure execution.

Mitral valve anatomy is complex, and one size does not fit all. More recently, percutaneous mitral valve interventions have revolutionized the management of primary and secondary mitral regurgitation (MR). However, edge-to-edge leaflet repair is not suitable for a large proportion of individuals including those with a failing bioprosthetic mitral valve/annuloplasty ring, and patients with significant mitral annular calcification resulting in mixed mitral valve disease/mitral stenosis. For this high risk cohort, transcatheter mitral valve replacement seems to be an attractive alternative.

Detailed preoperative and intraoperative echocardiographic assessment of the mitral valve apparatus is critical for a successful repair. The recent advent of 3-dimensional transesophageal echocardiography has added an extra pivotal role to transesophageal echocardiography in the assessment of mitral apparatus and mitral regurgitation. Because surgeons must rapidly decide whether cardiopulmonary bypass should be continued to be weaned off or a second pump run should be selected, the echocardiographer conducting intraoperative transesophageal echocardiography is required to be trained according to a certain algorithm. This review summarizes the current clinical role of intraoperative transesophageal echocardiography in mitral valve repair in the operating room.

Mitral valve disease is the most common valvular heart disease. Imaging determines the etiology (anatomic assessment), valve function and severity of valvular heart disease (hemodynamic assessment), remodeling of the left ventricle and right ventricle, and preplanning and guidance of percutaneous intervention. Although roles of computed tomography and magnetic resonance are increasing, echocardiography serves as the first-line imaging modality for the diagnosis and serial follow-up in most cases. This review summarizes the roles of multimodality imaging currently available from research fields to daily clinical practice.

Patients with heart failure often have mitral regurgitation, which can generate a vicious cycle. Medical therapy remains the cornerstone of their treatment in this setting. This review revisits the role of medical therapy and its optimization for severe functional mitral regurgitation in the contemporary era.

Transcatheter edge-to-edge mitral valve repair is a minimally invasive treatment option for selected patients with moderate to severe or severe mitral regurgitation. Although transcatheter edge-to-edge mitral valve repair offers a significant step forward in the management of mitral regurgitation, the rate of procedural-related complications is not trivial. High-quality periprocedural imaging is important for optimal patient selection and procedural success. In this review, we present a step-by-step approach of the recommended echocardiographic views for transcatheter edge-to-edge mitral valve repair.

Atrial functional mitral regurgitation (AFMR) can occur in patients with atrial fibrillation despite a preserved left ventricular systolic function. AFMR has received attention as a cause of heart failure; it is a therapeutic target in patients with heart failure with atrial fibrillation. Mitral annular dilatation from atrial fibrillation-induced left atrial dilatation is necessary for the generation of AFMR. Posterior mitral leaflet hamstringing also relates to the generation of AFMR. Further mitral annular dilatation owing to progressive left atrial and left ventricular dilatations, with mitral regurgitation-induced volume overload, worsens AFMR.

Mitral annular disjunction is a structural abnormality of the mitral annulus fibrosus, which has been described by pathologists to be associated with mitral leaflet prolapse. Mitral annular disjunction is a common finding in patients with myxomatous mitral valve diseases. The prevalence of mitral annular disjunction should be checked routinely during presurgical imaging. Otherwise, mitral annular disjunction itself might be an arrhythmogenic entity, irrespective of the presence of mitral valve prolapse (MVP). Therefore, we should check echocardiography keeping in mind mitral annular disjunction. Further prospective studies are needed to address whether a causative mechanistic link exists between mitral annular disjunction and arrhythmic MVP.

CARDIOLOGY CLINICS

SERIES OF RELATED INTEREST

Cardiac Electrophysiology Clinics
Available at: https://www.cardiacep.theclinics.com/
Heart Failure Clinics
Available at: https://www.heartfailure.theclinics.com/
Interventional Cardiology Clinics
Available at: https://www.interventional.theclinics.com/

THE CLINICS ARE AVAILABLE ONLINE!
Access your subscription at:
www.theclinics.com

Preface

Advances and Controversies in the Management of Mitral Valve Disease

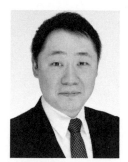

Takeshi Kitai, MD, PhD, FHFSA
Editor

Mitral regurgitation (MR) is among the most common valvular heart disorders. MR is classified as primary when it is due to a structural or degenerative abnormality of the valve, and secondary or functional MR occurs as a result of from left ventricular dysfunction or left atrial enlargement. While the surgical outcome has improved significantly over time for severe degenerative MR irrespective of symptoms, severe functional MR in patients with heart failure continues to be associated with poor outcomes from either ischemic or nonischemic cause. Determination of the mechanism of MR is paramount when formulating a treatment strategy because optimal management may differ depending on the underlying cause. Thus, a better understanding of the pathophysiology of each subset of patients with MR may have implications for treatment.

Despite recent advances in the catheter-based technologies, guideline-directed medical therapy (GDMT) remains the first-line management for symptomatic patients with MR, especially for functional MR. Although numerous nonrandomized studies have demonstrated high procedural success rates and good clinical outcomes with MitraClip repair in patients with symptomatic MR, the results of randomized controlled trial evaluating MitraClip repair versus GDMT are pending. In addition to the degenerative and functional MR, MR caused by infective endocarditis (IE) is the utmost important clinical entity.

The epidemiologic profile of IE has changed in recent decades, and early surgery is recommended in patients with complicated IE; however, its implementation in real-world clinical practice is still debated.

The overall goal of this special issue is to provide contemporary approaches and emerging surgical and interventional techniques in the evaluation and treatment of mitral valve disease. In this special issue, we would like to provide contemporary medical and diagnostic approaches, as well as emerging surgical and interventional techniques in the evaluation and treatment of mitral valve disease. The topics included in this special issue are advances in conventional surgical techniques, minimal invasive and robotic surgery and transcatheter mitral intervention in degenerative and functional MR, controversies regarding the timing of surgery in asymptomatic severe degenerative MR and active IE, and contemporary medical therapy directed at degenerative MR and functional MR in heart failure.

Takeshi Kitai, MD, PhD, FHFSA
Department of Cardiovascular Medicine
Kobe City Medical Center General Hospital
2-1-1 Minatojima-Minamimachi, Chuo-Ku
Kobe 6500047, Japan

E-mail address:
t-kitai@kcho.jp

cardiology.theclinics.com

Cardiol Clin 39 (2021) xi
https://doi.org/10.1016/j.ccl.2021.02.001
0733-8651/21/© 2021 Published by Elsevier Inc.

Advances in Mitral Valve Repair for Degenerative Mitral Regurgitation

Philosophy, Technical Details, and Long-Term Results

Benedetto Del Forno, MD*, Guido Ascione, MD, Michele De Bonis, MD

KEYWORDS

- Mitral regurgitation • Degenerative mitral valve disease • Barlow disease
- Myxomatous degeneration • Fibroelastic deficiency • Mitral valve repair • Centers of excellence
- Heart team

KEY POINTS

- Surgical mitral valve repair is the gold-standard treatment in severe degenerative mitral regurgitation.
- In patients with severe degenerative mitral regurgitation, timely surgical referral is crucial to achieve the best clinical outcome.
- A tImely surgical indication and an accurate application of the reparative techniques restore normal life expectancy and quality of life.
- Particularly in presence of complex lesions, patients should be referred to centers of excellence in order to maximize the likelihood as well as the durability of the repair.

INTRODUCTION

Mitral regurgitation (MR) is the second most frequent indication for heart valve surgery in the general population.[1–3]

In industrialized countries, myxomatous degeneration of the mitral leaflets[4] or fibroelastic deficiency[5] represent together the most common causes of primary MR reaching the 60% to 70% of all causes.[6]

In the first case, also known as Barlow disease, the valve surface is large, the leaflets are diffusely thick and distended resulting in a "floppy" aspect, and the chordae tendineae are elongated and occasionally broken. In addition, annular calcification of varying degrees as well as fibrosis and calcification of the papillary muscles may be observed. Those alterations are genetically transmitted.[7,8] Patients with Barlow disease are typically younger than 60 years with a long history of a regurgitant murmur.[9]

On the contrary, in case of "fibroelastic deficiency" the mitral valve is characterized by thin and translucent leaflets and the rupture of one or more chordae tendineae, usually those underlying the central portion of the posterior leaflet.[10] In many patients, an isolated myxomatous change of the prolapsing scallop may be observed. Patients with fibroelastic deficiency disease are typically older (>60 years) and present a short clinical

Conflict of interest: none to declare.
Department of Cardiac Surgery, Vita-Salute San Raffaele University, IRCCS San Raffaele Scientific Institute, Via Olgettina 60, Milan 20132, Italy
* Corresponding author.
E-mail address: delforno.benedetto@hsr.it

Cardiol Clin 39 (2021) 175–184
https://doi.org/10.1016/j.ccl.2021.01.001
0733-8651/21/© 2021 Elsevier Inc. All rights reserved.

history at the clinical presentation. Of note, the spectrum of variants between these 2 typical phenotypes is wide.

When left untreated, severe degenerative MR is associated with a high yearly mortality and incidence of cardiac events.[11,12] Conversely, a timely mitral valve repair is able to modify the poor natural history of these patients restoring a normal life expectancy, comparable to that of the age- and sex-matched general population.[13,14]

Alain Carpentier[15] developed and popularized reproducible mitral valve repair techniques, mostly based on resectional approaches, which have been adopted worldwide in the last 40 years. Likewise, Robert Frater[16] established the basis of a different way to repair the mitral valve by replacing native elongated or ruptured chordae tendineae, thus respecting the anatomy of the leaflets. In the recent years, both those methodologies have been increasingly used along with minimally invasive approaches and have confirmed their durability at long-term follow-up.

Particularly in Centers of Excellence for mitral valve repair, the innovations in cardiac imaging and the introduction of the Heart Team have further contributed to the refinement of the results based on a patient-tailored approach.

ECHOCARDIOGRAPHY: THE ESSENTIAL DIAGNOSTIC TOOL FOR MITRAL VALVE REPAIR

Transthoracic echocardiography is the most important diagnostic tool routinely used to evaluate the mitral valve anatomy, the mechanism, and the degree of MR as well as the dimensions and function of the cardiac chambers. Transesophageal echocardiography becomes essential whenever more accurate information is needed, especially for the planning of surgical or percutaneous interventions. The anatomy of the mitral valve apparatus, including leaflet, annulus, and subvalvular structures, should be always completely evaluated with the purpose to enable the detection of leaflet abnormalities (eg, thickness, redundancy, calcification), the presence of clefts, and/or annular calcifications.[17]

To further improve the diagnostic accuracy, a more realistic representation of the mitral valve complex is obtained by using 3-dimensional technology, which allows infinite possibilities of multiplanar reconstructions. Extremely precise details on clefts, gaps, and perforations of the leaflets or tissue deficiency are provided. In addition, acquirement of location of the flail, height of the prolapsing segment, length of the leaflets, precise position of the regurgitant jet, and distribution of

calcifications contribute to correctly plan the surgical procedure and decide on the repair technique. Finally, 3-dimensional echocardiography represents the gold standard to assess the mitral valve annular dimensions, guiding the selection of the prosthetic ring.

At the end of surgery, transesophageal echocardiography is key to assess the repair, detect any residual MR, and provide helpful details to refine the repair whenever necessary.[18]

EARLY REPAIR OR WATCHFUL WAITING: THE ROLE OF CENTERS OF EXCELLENCE

In the last few years, a significant increase in the number of patients submitted to mitral valve repair has been observed with a marked improvement of the outcomes and long-term results. Accordingly, the treatment of severe degenerative MR has been extended to asymptomatic patients in whom a successful and durable repair is very likely to be achieved with a very low operative risk.[19,20] Indeed, in patients with severe MR, symptoms may occur in a relatively advanced stage of the disease, when left ventricular dysfunction is already present and the surgical repair may not be able to restore normal life expectancy anymore.[21] On the other hand, asymptomatic patients without pulmonary hypertension, left ventricular dilatation, or dysfunction do have excellent postoperative outcomes.[11]

Those observations have been endorsed by both the European Society of Cardiology/European Association of Cardiothoracic Surgery and the American College of Cardiology/American Heart Association (ACC/AHA) guidelines, which advise mitral valve repair in asymptomatic patients with degenerative severe MR if the repair is performed in a center in which the likelihood of successful and durable repair exceeds 95% with an operative mortality risk of less than 1%.[22,23]

Nevertheless, it has to be emphasized that also the so called "watchful waiting" approach has been proposed and adopted in asymptomatic patients with severe degenerative MR with good results.[24] This strategy is based on the principle of postponing the operation until the onset of early symptoms or initial left ventricular dysfunction. When managed in an accurate manner, including active surveillance of the patients and serial echocardiographic examinations, this approach can also result in timely referral to surgery, excellent long-term survival, and good surgical outcomes.[25]

Although this matter remains the object of an ongoing debate, several groups have reported better outcomes with the "early repair" policy as compared with the "watchful waiting" approach, in terms of operative mortality, prevention of secondary atrial and ventricular remodeling, occurrence of atrial fibrillation, and functional tricuspid valve regurgitation.[11,20,26,27] Of course, the benefits of an early operation are completely related to a successful and durable repair. Moreover, an early repair policy has to be considered only if the surgical risk is very low. If those conditions are lacking, an early repair approach cannot be justified and advocated.[28]

The results of mitral valve repair can be highly variable worldwide. Although experienced groups report repair rates greater than 90% with an operative mortality less than 1%,[29,30] in real world practice, up to 50% of the patients still undergo mitral valve replacement, with the related higher operative mortality[31] and the exposure to prosthetic valve complications.[32]

The best outcomes are achieved by the so-called centers of excellence in mitral repair, where focused surgeons, cardiologists interested in mitral valve disease, and dedicated anesthesiologists strictly interact to build up and maintain a successful mitral valve repair program. Three main criteria are crucial to define a center of excellence: first of all, the annual volume of mitral repair procedures; secondly, expert periprocedural imaging capabilities; and finally, transparency regarding outcomes.[33]

The surgeons involved should perform at least 25 repairs per year, considering that an annual surgeon volume less than 25 operations was found to be associated with lower repair rate, higher 1-year mortality, and need of reoperation.[34,35]

Mitral valve repair surgery requires a significant learning curve strictly linked to the case-load of the center. Interestingly, a higher repair rate has been observed when low-volume surgeons work in high-volume centers.[35] This finding strongly confirms the weight of focused centers in which the patients are multidisciplinary managed and low-volume surgeons are mentored by the most experienced ones.

The accuracy of periprocedural imaging is also extremely important. At least one designated cardiologist with interest in mitral valve disease should be present in the team. Echocardiography must be routinely available and the obtained data should be audited for both quality control and education. Intraoperative transesophageal echocardiography performed by accredited anesthesiologists or cardiologists is crucial to guide and evaluate the repair. Finally, at discharge or at the first postoperative outpatient visit, an echocardiography should always be performed.

Core of a mitral valve repair center should be the transparency on the results. The goals of less than 1% mortality for isolated repair, a near 100% repair rate, and less than 5% failure rate at 5 years should be pursued, and the referring cardiologists should be correctly informed.

In addition, a reference center for mitral valve repair should be scientifically productive. A minimum number of 10 papers per year should be published on peer reviewed journals, and all the players of the center should be present as speakers at international meetings. Finally, the entire team should be always up-to-date on any new topic regarding this field,[34] and every innovative technique should be explored.[36]

SURGICAL MITRAL VALVE REPAIR
Objective

Mitral repair for degenerative MR aims to obtain a "neutralization" of the disease. A well-timed operation made before the onset of symptoms, atrial fibrillation, left ventricular dysfunction, or pulmonary hypertension can ensure a competent valve without stenosis, a preserved left ventricular function, the absence of arrhythmias, or significant concomitant tricuspid regurgitation. Once reached this goal, the patients will experience a survival expectancy similar to that of the general population.[13,37]

Timing of Mitral Regurgitation Correction

According to current European[22] and US[23] guidelines, mitral valve repair for primary MR is recommended in symptomatic patients or in those with left ventricular dysfunction. In asymptomatic patients with preserved left ventricular function, surgery should be considered in presence of pulmonary hypertension or atrial fibrillation. Surgery should also be considered in asymptomatic patients with preserved left ventricular ejection fraction ($\geq$60%) who are in sinus rhythm when left ventricular end-systolic diameter is greater than 40 mm according to the US guidelines or 40 to 44 mm for the European guidelines, when a durable mitral valve repair is likely and performed in a center of excellence and operative risk is low.

In the remaining asymptomatic patients, without other indication for surgery, the most appropriate management (early repair vs watchful waiting) remains controversial. However, in elderly patients with considerable comorbidities and/or complex valve lesions a "watchful waiting" approach seems more appropriate.[24]

Surgical Technique

In the last 20 years, an evolution of the reparative techniques and the surgical approaches has been progressively observed. As alternatives to conventional full median sternotomy, several mini-invasive approaches such as right minithoracotomy or totally endoscopic approach, with or without robotic assistance, have been increasingly used and preferred by many surgeons.

During mitral valve repair, an accurate exposure is key to perform the procedure. Left atriotomy through Waterstones groove remains the favorite approach to the mitral valve, although a transseptal incision or a superior approach through the roof of the left atrium may be adopted.

Once the mitral valve has been exposed, an in-depth analysis must be performed. In first instance, it is critical to discriminate between myxomatous degeneration and fibroelastic deficiency, and it is important to consider the possibilities of intermediate degrees between these 2 extreme forms. The mitral leaflets are gently pulled to assess their mobility and to identify chordal elongation or rupture. Because the anterior scallop of the posterior leaflet (P1) does not prolapse in most of the cases, it is commonly used as reference point to evaluate the presence and degree of prolapse of the other scallops of both leaflets. Subsequently, the subvalvular apparatus and the commissural area are assessed. Finally, the mitral annulus is checked to identify dilatation and calcification.

According to the classification proposed by Carpentier,[15] type II lesions are usually present in degenerative mitral valve pathology. The proper identification of those lesions will guide the choice of the reparative technique.

Aim of the repair approach, firstly described by Carpentier[15] and still largely adopted in the contemporary worldwide practice, is to restore the physiologic leaflets motion, to establish an adequate line of leaflets coaptation, and to stabilize the annulus.

Beside these concepts, new procedures have been proposed over the last years, including the use of artificial chordae[38] and the edge-to-edge technique.[39]

In the present days, greater than 95% of degenerative lesions can be successfully repaired in centers of excellence (**Table 1**).

PROSTHETIC ANNULAR RING

Prosthetic annuloplasty plays a key role in modern mitral valve repair and is routinely carried out using a ring or a band.

Table 1
Surgical mitral valve repair feasibility

	Easily Repairable Valve	Tough Anatomy	Relative Contraindications to Mitral Valve Repair
Involved leaflet	Posterior	Anterior or bileaflet	None
Leaflet calcifications	None	Mild	Moderate to severe
Annular calcifications	None	Mild to moderate	Severe or with significative leaflet involvement
Chordae tendineae and papillary muscles	Thin	Mild diffuse thickening	Severe and diffuse thickening with leaflet involvement
MR mechanism	Fibroelastic deficiency or focal myxomatous prolapse or flail	Forme fruste or bileaflet myxomatous disease. (Barlow); active or healed endocarditis with minimum leaflet destruction; mild leaflet fibrosis or thickening	Severe leaflet tethering or fibrosis; active or healed endocarditis with severe leaflet or annular tissue destruction
Adjunctive features	None	Mitral re-repair; anatomic context with high risk of systolic anterior motion; adult congenital pathologies	Mitral valve re-repair with little native leaflet tissue left; radiation-induced MR; papillary muscle rupture

The aim of prosthetic annuloplasty is to restore the normal shape of the annulus, the physiologic ratio between the anteroposterior and intercommissural annular diameters, to prevent further dilatation, and to increase the coaptation of the leaflets. All those effects strongly contribute to the long-term durability of the repair.[40–42]

POSTERIOR LEAFLET PROLAPSE
Triangular/Quadrangular Resection

The most frequent cause of degenerative MR is represented by the prolapse or flail of the central scallop (P2) of the posterior leaflet. When the lesion is very limited, a triangular resection of the prolapsing portion may be used (**Fig. 1**). Conversely, when the prolapse is relatively large, a quadrangular resection represents the technique of choice, eventually followed by plication of the annulus at the base of the resected portion.

However, annular plication may expose to the risk of kinking of the circumflex artery. A sliding or folding plasty can be alternatively adopted to avoid this complication and prevent a systolic anterior motion of the anterior leaflet by decreasing the height of the posterior mitral leaflet.

Artificial Chordae Implantation

Polytetrafluoroethylene (PTFE) chordal implantation has become a popular technique for the treatment of the prolapse or flail of the posterior leaflet. PTFE neochordae can be implanted in either anterior or posterior papillary muscles and then sutured to the free margin of the leaflet.

For the proper application of this technique, it is crucial to establish the correct length of PTFE neochordae. Different methods have been proposed, mostly consisting in adjusting the length of the neochordae after filling the left ventricle with saline or cardioplegia solution and then pushing the redundant leaflet tissue into the ventricle to obtain a good coaptation surface. Several years ago, modified artificial chordae with premeasured loops have been introduced to facilitate the use of this method. The proper length of the loop may be chosen preoperatively based on transesophageal echocardiography measurements or intraoperatively by using a dedicated caliper.

ANTERIOR LEAFLET PROLAPSE

The repair of anterior leaflet prolapse is more complex than the repair of the posterior one. Different techniques may be used.

Chordal Transfer

Chordal transfer consists in selecting the normal looking secondary chordae, detaching their insertion on the leaflet, and reattaching them to the margin of the anterior leaflet with 5.0 polypropylene suture. A limitation of this technique is the number of the normal chordae available in valves affected by extensive disease.

Chordal Transposition

Native normal chordae attached to the posterior leaflet can be transferred to the anterior one to correct a prolapsing segment.

The chosen chordae are resected from the posterior leaflet with a portion of the surrounding tissue and transposed on the free margin of the anterior leaflet.

A major advantage of this technique is that the transferred native chordae already have the correct length. Conversely, the main disadvantage is

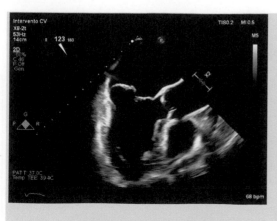
Pre-operative

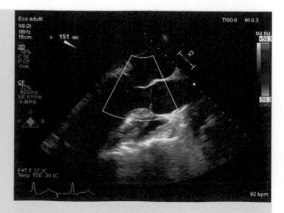
Post-operative

Fig. 1. Posterior leaflet prolapse treated by triangular resection.

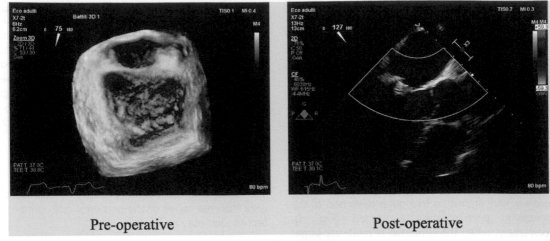

Pre-operative   Post-operative

Fig. 2. Anterior leaflet prolapse treated by neochordal implantation.

represented by the fact that a portion of the posterior leaflet not affected by the pathology will be resected.

Implantation of Artificial Chordae

The use of artificial PTFE neochordae is also indicated for the treatment of anterior leaflet prolapse (**Fig. 2**). The implantation technique, the measurement methods as well as the potential employment of preformed loops follow the same rules discussed for the disease of the posterior leaflet.

Edge-to-Edge Technique

A segmental prolapse of the anterior mitral valve leaflet can be effectively treated with the edge-to-edge technique. This technique consists of suturing together the matching edges of both leaflets at the site of MR. When the prolapse involves the

central scallop of the anterior leaflet (A2), this correction creates a double orifice valve. On the other hand, when the lateral (A1) or medial (A3) scallops of the anterior leaflet are affected by the prolapse, the edge-to-edge suture results in a single orifice valve with a relatively smaller area.

This approach allows a "functional" rather than an "anatomic" repair, which has nevertheless demonstrated an effectiveness and durability not inferior to conventional "anatomic repairs" at long-term.

BILEAFLET PROLAPSE

Simultaneous prolapse of both leaflets is typically observed in patients affected by global myxomatous degeneration of the mitral valve (Barlow disease). A combination of the surgical techniques previously described in the context of posterior

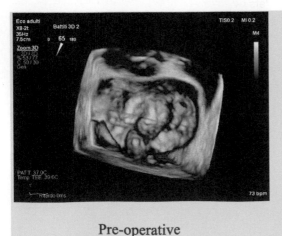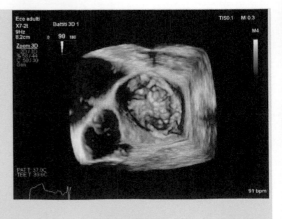

Pre-operative   Post-operative

Fig. 3. Bileaflet prolapse treated by edge-to-edge technique.

Table 2
Outcomes of mitral valve repair

	N. pts	30-d Mortality	Overall Survival	Freedom From/CI REDO	Freedom From/CI MR ≥3
Seeburger et al,[53] 2008	1339	2.4%	82.6% at 5 y	96.4% at 5 y	-
Di Bardino et al,[52] 2010	1042	0.6%	62% at 20 y	82% at 20 y	-
David et al,[50] 2013	606	0.8%	66.8 at 18 y	90.2 ± 2.4% at 18 y	67.5 ± 4.2% at 18 y
Yaffee et al,[49] 2014	1612	1.3%	77% (PB) 83% (CR)	95% (PB) 92% (CR)	91% (PB) 92% (CR)
Tabata et al,[48] 2014	700	1.3%	85.9% at 12 y	88.7% at 12 y	72.3% at 12 y
Coutinho et al,[37] 2016	475	1.2%	61 ± 3.7% at 15 y	88 ± 2.7 at 20 y	-
Suri et al,[42] 2016	1218	-	-	6.9 ± 1% at 15 y	13.3 ± 1.2% at 15 y
Li et al,[54] 2020	322	1.6%	96.9%	91.2	73.4%

Abbreviations: CI, cumulative incidence; CR, complete ring; PB, posterior band.

and anterior leaflet prolapse can be used to address the multiple lesions characteristic of this etiology. Alternatively, the edge-to-edge technique dose have one of its best indications in this difficult setting (**Fig. 3**).

RESULTS OF SURGERY

Despite the absence of randomized trials, all the observational data accumulated so far have demonstrated that mitral valve repair is associated with lower hospital mortality, better survival, and lower morbidity at long-term as compared with mitral valve replacement.[43] Remarkably, in degenerative mitral valve disease, hospital mortality after isolated mitral valve repair is less than 1% in high-volume centers.[44–46]

Patients undergoing mitral valve repair before the onset of symptoms and left ventricular dysfunction will experience survival and quality of life similar to that of the same-age healthy general population.[13,37] Conversely, life expectancy will be significantly decreased if the procedure is carried out in patients with reduced LVEF or with symptoms of congestive heart failure.[47]

The long-term durability of mitral valve repair depends on the lesions causing the regurgitation, the surgical technique, and the experience of the center. The presence of residual MR greater than mild immediately after surgery is a strong predictor of repair failure at long term.

In many studies, the long-term durability of mitral repair is still evaluated by using the freedom from reoperation. Nowadays this cannot be

considered an accurate parameter because the reoperation rate underscores the true recurrence of MR, which should represent the only endpoint to assess the validity of the repair technique[42,46,48–50] (**Table 2**).

Different results have been observed according to the involved leaflet. For the isolated prolapse of the posterior leaflet, both freedom from reoperation and freedom from recurrence of moderate or severe MR are excellent, especially when surgery is performed in high-volume center.

Conversely, for anterior and in bileaflet prolapse, the outcomes in terms of rate of recurrence of moderate or severe MR are less favorable, with this risk approaching 1% to 2% per year.[48–53]

The presence of annular calcification, large leaflets prolapse in the context of severe myxomatous degeneration, and subvalvular involvement are some of the conditions that make the repair particularly challenging.

Specifically, in these complex cases, patients should be referred to experienced centers with a multidisciplinary heart team to maximize the likelihood of a durable reconstruction.[34]

SUMMARY

Surgical mitral valve repair represents the standard of care for patients with severe degenerative MR. This approach is safe and almost invariably feasible, especially when performed in high-volume centers. A timely surgical referral is crucial to carry out the operation with a very low operative risk. In addition, using the appropriate techniques, the durability of mitral valve repair is excellent, and normal life expectancy combined with good quality of life is restored.

CLINICS CARE POINTS

- Patients with severe degenerative mitral regurgitation left untreated show a poor clinical outcome.
- Appropriate surgical correction of mitral regurgitation provides a restored life expectancy and quality of life.
- Heart Team approach and centers of excellence for mitral valve repair are important to obtain a durable valve repair with low surgical risk.

COMPETING INTERESTS

The authors declare no competing interests.

REFERENCE

1. Delling FN, Rong J, Larson MG, et al. Evolution of mitral valve prolapse: insights from the framingham heart study. Circulation 2016;133(17):1688–95.
2. Nkomo VT, Gardin JM, Skelton TN, et al. Burden of valvular heart diseases: a population-based study. Lancet 2006;368(9540):1005–11.
3. D'Arcy JL, Coffey S, Loudon MA, et al. Large-scale community echocardiographic screening reveals a major burden of undiagnosed valvular heart disease in older people: the OxVALVE Population Cohort Study. Eur Heart J 2016;37(47):3515–22.
4. Barlow J, Pocock W. The significance of late systolic murmurs and mid-late systolic clicks. Am Heart J 1963;66:443.
5. Mills WR, Barber JE, Ratliff NB, et al. Biomechanical and echocardiographic characterization of flail mitral leaflet due to myxomatous disease: further evidence for early surgical intervention. Am Heart J 2004;148:144–50.
6. Olson L, Subramanian R, Ackermann D, et al. Surgical pathology of the mitral valve: a study of 712 cases spanning 21 years. Mayo Clin Proc 1987;62: 22–34.
7. Disse S, Abergel E, Berrebi A, et al. Mapping of a first locus for autosomal dominant myxomatous mitral-valve prolapse to chromosome 16p11.2–p12.1. Am J Hum Genet 1999;65:1242–51.
8. Trochu JN, Kyndt F, Schott JJ, et al. Clinical characteristics of a familial inherited myxomatous valvular

dystrophy mapped to Xq28. J Am Coll Cardiol 2000;35:1890–7.
9. Carpentier AF, Pellerin M, Fuzellier JF, et al. Extensive calcification of the mitral valve anulus: pathology and surgical management. J Thorac Cardiovasc Surg 1996;111:718–29.
10. Carpentier A, Lacour-Gayet F, Camilleri J. Fibroelastic dysplasia of the mitral valve: an anatomical and clinical entity. Circulation 1982;3:307.
11. Enriquez-Sarano M, Avierinos JF, Messika-Zeitoun D, et al. Quantitative determinants of the outcome of asymptomatic mitral regurgitation. N Engl J Med 2005;352:875–83.
12. Ling H, Enriquez-Sarano M, Seward J, et al. Clinical outcome of mitral regurgitation due to flail leaflets. N Engl J Med 1996;335:1417–23.
13. Watt TMF, Brescia AA, Murray SL, et al. Degenerative mitral valve repair restores life expectancy. Ann Thorac Surg 2020;109:794–801.
14. Vassileva CM, Mishkel G, McNeely C, et al. Long-term survival of patients undergoing mitral valve repair and replacement: a longitudinal analysis of Medicare fee-for-service beneficiaries. Circulation 2013;127(18):1870–6.
15. Carpentier A. Cardiac valve surgery — the 'French correction'. J Thorac Cardiovasc Surg 1983;86(3): 323–37.
16. Frater RWM. Anatomical rules for the plastic repair of a diseased mitral valve. Thorax 1964;19:458–64.
17. Zoghbi WA, Adams D, Bonow RO, et al. Recommendations for noninvasive evaluation of native valvular regurgitation: a report from the American Society of Echocardiography developed in collaboration with the Society for Cardiovascular Magnetic Resonance. J Am Soc Echocardiogr 2017;30(4):303–71.
18. De Bonis M, Alfieri O, Dalrymple-Hay M, et al. Mitral valve repair in degenerative mitral regurgitation: state of the art. Prog Cardiovasc Dis 2017;60(3): 386–93.
19. Adams DH, Anyanwu AC, Rahmanian PB, et al. Current concepts in mitral valve repair for degenerative disease. Heart Fail Rev 2006;11:241–57.
20. Kang DH, Kim JH, Rim JH, et al. Comparison of early surgery versus conventional treatment in asymptomatic severe mitral regurgitation. Circulation 2009; 119:797–804.
21. Tribouilloy CM, Enriquez-Sarano M, Schaff HV, et al. Impact of preoperative symptoms on survival after surgical correction of organic mitral regurgitation: rationale for optimizing surgical indications. Circulation 1999;99(3):400–5.
22. Baumgartner H, Falk V, Bax JJ, et al. 2017 ESC/ EACTS guidelines for the management of valvular heart disease. Eur Heart J 2017;38(36):2739–91.
23. Nishimura RA, Otto CM, Bonow RO, et al. 2017 AHA/ ACC focused Update of the 2014 AHA/ACC guideline for the management of patients with valvular

heart disease: a report of the American College of Cardiology/American Heart Association Task Force on clinical practice guidelines. irculation 2017; 135(25):e1159–95.

24. Rosenhek R, Rader F, Klaar U, et al. Outcome of watchful waiting in asymptomatic severe mitral regurgitation. Circulation 2006;113:2238–44.

25. Zilberszac R, Heinze G, Binder T, et al. Long-term outcome of active surveillance in severe but asymptomatic primary mitral regurgitation. JACC Cardiovasc Imaging 2018;11(9):1213–21.

26. Montant P, Chenot F, Robert A, et al. Long-term survival in asymptomatic patients with severe degenerative mitral regurgitation: a propensity score-based comparison between an early surgical strategy and a conservative treatment approach. J Thorac Cardiovasc Surg 2009;138(6):1339–48.

27. Yazdchi F, Koch CG, Mihaljevic T, et al. Increasing disadvantage of "watchful waiting" for repairing degenerative mitral valve disease. Ann Thorac Surg 2015;99(6):1992–2000.

28. De Bonis M, Bolling SF. Mitral valve surgery: wait and see vs. early operation. Eur Heart J 2013; 34(1):13–19a.

29. Gillinov AM, Mihaljevic T, Blackstone EH, et al. Should patients with severe degenerative mitral regurgitation delay surgery until symptoms develop? Ann Thorac Surg 2010;90(2):481–8.

30. Castillo JG, Anyanwu AC, Fuster V, et al. A near 100% repair rate for mitral valve prolapse is achievable in a reference center: implications for future guidelines. J Thorac Cardiovasc Surg 2012;144(2): 308–12.

31. Bolling SF, Li S, O'Brien SM, et al. Predictors of mitral valve repair: clinical and surgeon factors. Ann Thorac Surg 2010;90:1904–11.

32. Jung JC, Jang MJ, Hwang HY. Meta-analysis comparing mitral valve repair versus replacement for degenerative mitral regurgitation across all ages. Am J Cardiol 2019;123(3):446–53.

33. Bonow RO, Adams DH. The time has come to define centers of excellence in mitral valve repair. J Am Coll Cardiol 2016;67(5):499–501.

34. Bridgewater B, Hooper T, Munsch C, et al. Mitral repair best practice: proposed standards. Heart 2006;92:939–44.

35. Chikwe J, Toyoda N, Anyanwu AC, et al. Relation of mitral valve surgery volume to repair rate, durability, and survival. J Am Coll Cardiol 2017. https://doi.org/ 10.1016/j.jacc.2017.02.026 [pii:S0735-1097(17) 30677-0].

36. Del Forno B, De Bonis M, Agricola E, et al. Mitral valve regurgitation: a disease with a wide spectrum of therapeutic options. Nat Rev Cardiol 2020. https:// doi.org/10.1038/s41569-020-0395-7.

37. Coutinho GF, Correia PM, Branco C, et al. Long-term results of mitral valve surgery for degenerative anterior leaflet or bileaflet prolapse: analysis of negative factors for repair, early and late failures, and survival. Eur J Cardiothorac Surg 2016;50(1):66–74.

38. Bortolotti U, Milano AD, Frater RW. Mitral valve repair with artificial chordae: a review of its history, technical details, long- term results, and pathology. Ann Thorac Surg 2012;93(2):684–91.

39. Alfieri O, Maisano F. An effective technique to correct anterior mitral leaflet prolapse. J Card Surg 1999;14(6):468–70.

40. Gillinov AM, Cosgrove DM, Blackstone EH, et al. Durability of mitral valve repair for degenerative disease. J Thorac Cardiovasc Surg 1998;116(5): 734–43.

41. David TE, Armstrong S, McCrindle BW, et al. Late outcomes of mitral valve repair for mitral regurgitation due to degenerative disease. Circulation 2013; 127(14):1485–92.

42. Suri RM, Clavel MA, Schaff HV, et al. Effect of recurrent mitral regurgitation following degenerative mitral valve repair: long-term analysis of competing outcomes. J Am Coll Cardiol 2016;67:488–98.

43. Lazam S, Vanoverschelde JL, Tribouilloy C, et al. MIDA (Mitral Regurgitation International Database) Investigators. Twenty-year outcome after mitral repair versus replacement for severe degenerative mitral regurgitation: analysis of a large, prospective, multicenter, international registry. Circulation 2017; 135(5):410–22.

44. Castillo JG, Anyanwu AC, El-Eshmawi A, et al. All anterior and bileaflet mitral valve prolapses are repairable in the modern era of reconstructive surgery. Eur J Cardiothorac Surg 2014;45(1): 139–45.

45. Gammie JS, O'Brien SM, Griffith BP, et al. Influence of hospital procedural volume on care process and mortality for patients undergoing elective surgery for mitral regurgitation. Circulation 2007;115(7): 881–7.

46. De Bonis M, Lapenna E, Taramasso M, et al. Very long-term durability of the edge- to-edge repair for isolated anterior mitral leaflet prolapse: up to 21 years of clinical and echocardiographic results. J Thorac Cardiovasc Surg 2014;148(5): 2027–32.

47. Detaint D, Sundt TM, Nkomo VT, et al. Surgical correction of mitral regurgitation in the elderly: outcomes and recent improvements. Circulation 2006; 114(4):265–72.

48. Tabata M, Kasegawa H, Fukui T, et al. Long-term outcomes of artificial chordal replacement with tourniquet technique in mitral valve repair: a single-center experience of 700 cases. J Thorac Cardiovasc Surg 2014;148(5):2033–8.

49. Yaffee DW, Loulmet DF, Zias EA, et al. Long-term results of mitral valve repair with semi-rigid posterior

band annuloplasty. J Heart Valve Dis 2014;23(1): 66–71.

50. David TE, Armstrong S, Ivanov J. Chordal replacement with polytetrafluoroethylene sutures formitral valve repair: a 25-years experience. J Thorac Cardiovasc Surg 2013;145:1563–9.

51. Braunberger E, Deloche A, BerrebiA, et al. Very long-term results (more than 20 years) of valve repair with carpentier's techniques in nonrheumatic mitral valve insufficiency. Circulation 2001;104(12 Suppl 1):I8–11.

52. Di Bardino DJ, ElBardissi AW, McClure RS, et al. Four decades of experience with mitral valve repair: analysis of differential indications, technical evolution, and long-term outcome. J Thorac Cardiovasc Surg 2010;139(1):76–83.

53. Seeburger J, Borger MA, Falk V, et al. Minimal invasive mitral valve repair for mitral regurgitation: results of 1339 consecutive patients. Eur J Cardiothorac Surg 2008;34(4):760–5.

54. Li J, Zhao Y, Zhou T, et al. Mitral valve repair for degenerative mitral regurgitation in patients with left ventricular systolic dysfunction: early and mid-term outcomes. J Cardiothorac Surg 2020; 15:284.

The Role of Surgical Treatment of Severe Functional Mitral Regurgitation in Heart Failure

Khalil Fattouch, MD, PhD*, Francesco Guccione, MD, PhD

KEYWORDS

• Mitral valve • Secondary regurgitation • Surgical options • Transcatheter therapy

KEY POINTS

- Patient selection is mandatory to successful mitral valve repair in functional mitral valve regurgitation.
- Preoperative echo evaluation is critical to better evaluate the anatomic modification of the mitral apparatus.
- In light of recent randomized trials, several patients could benefit from transcatheter mitral therapy.
- Mitral annuloplasty is not effective in all patients with functional mitral valve regurgitation; meanwhile, adding surgical techniques should be performed to improve the repair durability.

INTRODUCTION

Functional mitral regurgitation (FMR) is a common clinical entity that will likely increase in the future due to predicted demographic changes. It is also associated with poor long-term survival. The anatomic structure of the mitral valve apparatus is complex and consists of several components, each of which can be affected by a variety of diseases resulting in mitral regurgitation (MR).

In primary MR, the valvular incompetence is caused by compromised or structurally disrupted components of the valve apparatus.

In secondary or FMR, the mitral apparatus is structurally normal, with the regurgitation resulting from failure of coaptation of the mitral valve leaflets without coexisting structural changes of the valve itself.

As a consequence of this, we see a systolic retrograde flow from the left ventricle into the left atrium due to reduction of the normal systolic coaptation of the mitral valve leaflets. A slow progression of the symptoms is typical for this valve disease and often ends in irreversible left ventricular dysfunction.

The pathophysiology and treatment of FMR are quite complex.

Given the complexity of its pathogenesis, a solution to correct the valvular and subvalvular dysfunction, along with the left ventricular (LV) geometric distortion associated with ischemic MR (IMR) has not yet been elucidated.[1,2]

DEFINITION OF SEVERE FUNCTIONAL MITRAL REGURGITATION

In the 2017 European Society of Cardiology (ESC) guidelines, an effective regurgitant orifice area (EROA) ≥ 20 mm^2 and a regurgitant volume (RV) ≥ 30 mL are considered as cutoff values to define severe FMR,[3] whereas in the 2017 American College of Cardiology/American Heart Association (ACC/AHA) guideline update severe FMR, similarly to severe primary MR, is defined as an EROA ≥ 40 mm^2 and an RV ≥ 60 mL.[4] Current divergences between European and American recommendations confirm that assessment of FMR severity is challenging for several reasons.

Department of Cardiovascular Surgery, GVM Care and Research, Maria Eleonora Hospital, Viale Regione Siciliana 1571, Palermo 90100, Italy
* Corresponding author.
E-mail address: khalilfattouch@hotmail.com

Cardiol Clin 39 (2021) 185–188
https://doi.org/10.1016/j.ccl.2021.01.012

1. First, lower EROAs (≥ 20 mm^2 vs ≥ 40 mm^2) have been shown to be associated with a worse prognosis in patients with FMR compared with those affected by primary MR.
2. Second, EROA may be underestimated in patients with FMR due to its semilunar instead of round shape, as in primary MR.
3. Third, in the presence of LV dysfunction and low stroke volume, smaller RVs reflect a significant regurgitation fraction.
4. Finally, FMR is a dynamic condition and its degree may change depending on the phase of cardiac cycle and loading conditions (ie, systemic arterial pressure, medical therapy, exercise). Exercise echocardiography can play a crucial role in the assessment and quantification of the dynamic component of FMR.[5]

Importantly, FMR severity should always be evaluated after optimization of guideline-directed medical therapy (GDMT). Finally, clinical and echocardiographic findings should be integrated to prevent unnecessary intervention when MR may not be as severe as documented on noninvasive studies.

CURRENT GUIDELINES
In Accordance with American Heart Association Guidelines

Class I

1. Patients with chronic secondary MR (stages B to D) and heart failure (HF) with reduced LV ejection fraction (LVEF) should receive standard GDMT therapy for HF, including angiotensin-converting enzyme inhibitors, angiotensin receptor blockers, beta blockers, and/or aldosterone antagonists as indicated. (Level of Evidence: A)
2. Cardiac resynchronization therapy with biventricular pacing is recommended for symptomatic patients with chronic severe secondary MR (stages B to D) who meet the indications for device therapy

Class IIa

1. Mitral valve surgery is reasonable for patients with chronic severe secondary MR (stages C and D) who are undergoing coronary artery bypass grafting (CABG) or aortic valve replacement. (Level of Evidence: C)

Class IIb

- Mitral valve repair or replacement may be considered for severely symptomatic patients (New York Heart Association [NYHA] class III to IV) with chronic severe secondary MR (stage D) who have persistent symptoms despite optimal GDMT for HF. (Level of Evidence: B)
- Mitral valve repair may be considered for patients with chronic moderate secondary MR (stage B) who are undergoing other cardiac surgery. (Level of Evidence: C)

In According with European Society of Cardiology Guidelines

I C

Surgery is indicated in patients with severe secondary MR undergoing CABG and LVEF greater than 30%.

II A C

Surgery should be considered in symptomatic patients with severe secondary MR, LVEF less than 30% but with an option for revascularization and evidence of myocardial viability.

II B C

- When revascularization is not indicated, surgery may be considered in patients with severe secondary MR and LVEF greater than 30% who remain symptomatic despite optimal medical management (including cardiac resynchronization therapy [CRT] if indicated) and have a low surgical risk.
- When revascularization is not indicated and surgical risk is not low, a percutaneous edge-to-edge procedure may be considered in patients with severe secondary MR and LVEF greater than 30% who remain symptomatic despite optimal medical management (including CRT if indicated) and who have a suitable valve morphology by echocardiography, avoiding futility.
- In patients with severe secondary MR and LVEF less than 30% who remain symptomatic despite optimal medical management (including CRT if indicated) and who have no option for revascularization, the heart team may consider a percutaneous edge-to-edge procedure or valve surgery after careful evaluation for a ventricular assist device or heart transplantation according to individual patient characteristics.

It therefore appears evident that the role of mitral valve surgery for the treatment of isolated severe FMR is also unclear. European recommendations suggest surgical treatment in this scenario only for patients with severe HF symptoms despite optimal GDMT, LVEF greater than 30%, and low comorbidity burden.

SURGICAL TREATMENT OF FUNCTIONAL MITRAL REGURGITATION

The most commonly recommended surgery for patients with moderate or severe FMR is mitral valve repair or chordal sparing replacement, but a lack of conclusive evidence in favor of one or the other technique has left the choice largely to the surgeon's preference and expertise. Several randomized and observational studies have found that restrictive mitral valve repair is associated with lower perioperative mortality but has high rate of MR recurrence, which is cited at 30% to 60% at mid-term follow-up.[6,7] Undersizing valve repair is preferentially performed with closed rings, often with predetermined geometry, compared with partial ring or band. Conversely, replacement provides better long-term correction with a lower risk of MR recurrence and repeat surgery but has higher perioperative morbidity. A recent meta-analysis reported a rate of death at 35% higher in the replacement patients than in the repair subjects. This relative long-term risk has been attributed to the fact that patients undergoing mitral valve replacement tend to be older and have more coexisting illnesses than those undergoing repair.[8] Complete preservation of subvalvular apparatus is recommended.

The mitral valve repair technique most commonly performed is a restrictive annuloplasty with the use of a rigid or semirigid ring to downsize the annulus diameter. Combined restrictive annuloplasty and subvalvular procedures directly addressing papillary muscle (PM) displacement and leaflet tethering also have been successfully performed.

Procedures involving the PMs require knowledge of their anatomy and blood flow distribution, as well as recognition of the different divisions of PMs and anatomic variants. Two main procedures are performed in this context: PM approximation or "sling," and PM relocation.

TRANSCATHETER THERAPY

Percutaneous MR treatment mimics surgery by using annuloplasty, edge-to-edge repair, or prosthesis implantation.

Reduction of the severity of MR may be accomplished percutaneously by approximation of the anterior and posterior mitral leaflets, a procedure that leads to formation of a double-orifice valve. In the randomized Endovascular Valve Edge-to-Edge Repair Study (EVEREST) II, transcatheter mitral-leaflet approximation with the MitraClip device (Abbott, Chicago, IL) was safer than surgical mitral valve repair but was not as effective in reducing the severity of MR.

It should be noted, however, that patients included in EVEREST II were low-risk candidates for surgery mainly affected by primary MR (73.4%), and, hence, quite different from those undergoing MitraClip treatment in current practice in Europe.

For many years after the publication of EVEREST II results, evidence supporting the use of MitraClip for the treatment of FMR was derived only from observational studies.

Recently, 2 intensely awaited randomized controlled trials have been published. Both MITRA-FR (Multicentre Study of Percutaneous Mitral Valve Repair MitraClip Device in Patients With Severe Secondary Mitral Regurgitation) and COAPT (Cardiovascular Outcomes Assessment of the MitraClip Percutaneous Therapy for Heart Failure Patients with Functional Mitral Regurgitation) investigated the role of MitraClip treatment in patients with ischemic or nonischemic FMR, who remained symptomatic (NYHA class II–IV) despite GDMT.[9,10]

In COAPT, device-based treatment resulted in a significantly lower rate of hospitalization for HF, lower mortality, and better quality of life and functional capacity within 24 months of follow-up than medical therapy alone. In addition, the rate of freedom from device-related complications with transcatheter mitral valve repair exceeded a pre-specified objective performance goal.

A total of 614 patients with moderate-to-severe (3+) or severe (4+) FMR (EROA >30 mm^2 and RV >45 mL), NYHA class II–IV, and LVEF 20% to 50% were randomized to MitraClip plus GDMT (n = 302) or GDMT alone (n = 312). The primary effectiveness endpoint (HF hospitalizations at 24 months) was significantly lower in the MitraClip group compared with the GDMT group (35.8% vs 67.9% per patient-year; hazard ratio [HR]0.53, 95% confidence interval [CI] 0.40–0.70; P<.001) with a very favorable number needed to treat of 3.1. Importantly, significant differences between groups were also observed in the composite of death and HF hospitalization at 1 year (45.7% in the device arm vs 67.9% in the control arm; HR 0.57, 95% CI 0.45–0.72; P<.001), all-cause mortality alone at 24 months (29.1% in the device arm vs 46.1% in the control arm; HR 0.62, 95% CI 0.46–0.82), and need for LV assist device at 1 year (3% in the device arm vs 7.1% in the control arm; HR 0.34, 95% CI 0.13–0.87; P = .02).

In the MITRA-FR trial, 6304 patients with severe FMR (defined as EROA >20 mm^2 and RV >30 mL), NYHA class II–IV, and LVEF 15% to 40%, were randomized to MitraClip plus GDMT (n = 152) or GDMT alone (n = 152). The primary composite endpoint (all-cause death and hospitalization for HF at 12 months) was similar between the 2 arms (54.6% in the device group vs 51.3% in the control group; odds ratio 1.16, 95% CI 0.73–1.84), and both single endpoints did not significantly differ between groups. No significant differences were noted across specified subgroups.

SUMMARY

In conclusion, it appears there is no agreement between the 2 trials; however, we think that the results of MITRA-FR and COAPT trials should be interpreted as complementary rather than contradictory.

To obtain a prognostic benefit, only selected patients should receive MitraClip therapy. Accurate evaluation of GDMT before intervention is essential. GDMT is also necessary after the intervention. This reinforces the importance of the heart team with active participation of HF specialists in decision making and patient management. Intervention should be considered only in the presence of severe FMR, defined as EROA >30 mm^2 and RV >45 mL according to COAPT criteria. Finally, it is important to exclude patients with advanced cardiomyopathy, defined as NYHA class IV, right ventricular failure, severe tricuspid regurgitation, as well as patients with marked LV dilatation or severely reduced LVEF. In these patients, LV assist device/transplantation should be discussed by the heart team if appropriate, whereas patients in whom no benefit could be expected from any intervention should stay on GDMT.

Percutaneous intervention (ie, MitraClip), when used in a timely manner in properly selected patients, may interrupt the vicious circle that ultimately leads to end-stage HF in patients with chronic HF.

CLINICS CARE POINTS

- Patient selection and preoperative echocardiographic evaluation are critical for successful mitral valve repair in functional mitral regurgitation.
- Transcatheter mitral valve intervention would be beneficial in selected patients with functional mitral regurgitation.
- Mitral annuloplasty alone is not effective in some patients, and additional surgical techniques should be considered to improve the repair durability.

DISCLOSURE

The authors have nothing to disclose.

REFERENCES

1. Nappi F, Spadaccio C, Nenna A, et al. Is subvalvular repair worthwhile in severe ischemic mitral regurgitation? Subanalysis of the papillary muscle approximation trial. J Thorac Cardiovasc Surg 2017;153:286–95.e2.

2. Timek TA. Sub or snub: is subvalvular repair worthwhile in severe ischemic mitral regurgitation? J Thorac Cardiovasc Surg 2017;153:296–7.

3. Baumgartner H, Falk V, Bax JJ, et al. 2017 ESC/EACTS guidelines for the management of valvular heart disease. Eur Heart J 2017;38:2739–91.

4. Nishimura RA, Otto CM, Bonow RO, et al. AHA/ACC focused update of the 2014 AHA/ACC guideline for the management of patients with valvular heart disease: a report of the American College of Cardiology/American Heart Association Task Force on Clinical Practice Guidelines. Circulation 2017;135: e1159–95.

5. Zoghbi WA, Adams D, Bonow RO, et al. Recommendations for noninvasive evaluation of native valvular regurgitation: a report from the American Society of Echocardiography developed in collaboration with the Society for Cardiovascular Magnetic Resonance. J Am Soc Echocardiogr 2017;30:303–71.

6. Acker MA, Parides MK, Perrault LP, et al. Mitral-valve repair versus replacement for severe ischemic mitral regurgitation. N Engl J Med 2014;370:23–32.

7. Goldstein D, Moskowitz AJ, Gelijns AC, et al. Two-year outcomes of surgical treatment of severe ischemic mitral regurgitation. N Engl J Med 2016; 374:344–53.

8. Vassileva CM, Boley T, Markwell S, et al. Meta-analysis of short-term and long-term survival following repair versus replacement for ischemic mitral regurgitation. Eur J Cardiothorac Surg 2011;39: 295–303.

9. Obadia JF, Messika-Zeitoun D, Leurent G, et al, MITRA-FR Investigators. Percutaneous repair or medical treatment for secondary mitral regurgitation. N Engl J Med 2018;379:2297–306.

10. Stone GW, Lindenfeld J, Abraham WT, et al, COAPT Investigators. Transcatheter mitral-valve repair in patients with heart failure. N Engl J Med 2018;379: 2307–18.

Role of Mitral Valve Repair for Mitral Infective Endocarditis

Yukikatsu Okada, MD, PhD[a,*], Takeo Nakai, MD[a], Takeshi Kitai, MD, PhD[b]

KEYWORDS

- Mitral valve infective endocarditis • Mitral valve repair • Autologous pericardium • Ring annuloplasty
- Mitral valve replacement

KEY POINTS

- Systematic reviews and meta-analyses have demonstrated that mitral valve repair (MVrep), whenever feasible, yields better short- and long-term outcomes than mitral valve replacement in the treatment of mitral infective endocarditis (IE).
- The key factors determining reparability are the extent and location of tissue destruction by the endocarditic process and the quality of the remaining tissue after radical resection of infected tissue.
- MVrep, using a wide armamentarium of reparative procedures, has the potential to improve late outcomes in patients undergoing mitral valve surgery for mitral IE. Early repair-oriented surgery is recommended for mitral IE.

 Video content accompanies this article at http://www.cardiology.theclinics.com.

INTRODUCTION

Mitral valve replacement (MVR) using mechanical or bioprosthetic valves was the standard procedure for mitral valve infective endocarditis (IE) until the publication of the initial series on mitral valve repair (MVrep) for acute endocarditis by Dreyfus and colleagues[1] in 1990. They reported 40 patients undergoing MVrep for acute mitral IE using several reparative techniques including the pericardial patch technique as a leaflet substitute. The development of new techniques allowed them to increase their repair rate up to 80% without recurrence of endocarditis or reoperation for valvular insufficiency. Muehrcke reported 146 patients undergoing surgery for mitral IE.[2] MVrep was accomplished in 70% of the patients with lower hospital mortality and improved long-term survival.

Although only a limited number of studies focusing on MVrep for IE were available until 2000, clinical evidence suggesting improved outcomes with MVrep for mitral IE during the last 2 decades has increased. The principal concern is the impact of active infection on the feasibility and durability of repair. To avoid recurrence of infection, chordal reconstruction using chordal transport or annulus reinforcement without a prosthetic ring was advised in the early stages. Systematic reviews and meta-analyses have demonstrated that MVrep, whenever feasible, yields better short-term and long-term results than replacement in the treatment of mitral IE.[3,4] The feasibility of repair depends on the extent of destruction of the mitral valve and the surgeon's experience. The guidelines[5–7] recommend MVrep, whenever possible, for patients with mitral IE. The aim of this review was to summarize the history, reliable repair

[a] Heart Valve Center, Midori Hospital, 1-16 Edayoshi Nishi-ku, Kobe 651-2133, Japan; [b] Department of Cardiovascular Medicine, Kobe City Medical Center General Hospital, 2-1-1 Minatojimaminamimachi Chuo-ku, Kobe 650-0047, Japan
* Corresponding author.
E-mail address: yukikatsuok@gmail.com

Cardiol Clin 39 (2021) 189–196
https://doi.org/10.1016/j.ccl.2021.01.005
0733-8651/21/

procedures, and clinical results of MVrep for mitral IE to ensure improved event-free survival rates after surgery.

METHODS

A search of the PubMed database was conducted for articles published from January 2000 to July 2020. Pertinent articles were selected using the following keywords: "mitral valve repair," "infective endocarditis," and "late results." Only articles in English and involving human subjects were included. Case reports, small case series with fewer than 30 cases of MVrep, or studies with missing surgical details were excluded. When more than one study had been published by a particular center, only the most recent study with the largest number of patients was included in this review.

RESULTS

Reports on Mitral Valve Repair for Infective Endocarditis in the 1990s

There were only 4 studies on MVrep for mitral IE from 1990 to 1999.[1,2,8,9] First, Dreyfus and colleagues reported a series of 40 patients with a mean follow-up of 30 months who had undergone MVrep for acute endocarditis in 1990. They stated that the organisms involved must not influence the surgical policy. The only factor limiting valve repair in IE, they believed, was the extent of the lesions. The entire anterior leaflet of the mitral valve was replaced with pericardium in 3 patients. A procedure of this kind was only possible when the infectious process did not involve the marginal chordae. Preservation of the marginal chordae is an important procedure. Barring such cases, chordal transposition was considered mandatory in all cases of ruptured chordae of the anterior leaflet. The repair rate was 80% using Carpentier's reconstructive techniques, including the use of pericardial patches.[10] They concluded that valve repair in acute endocarditis is possible and effective in most cases. Pagani and colleagues[8] reported a series of 22 patients with a mean follow-up of 20 months; there were no cases of recurrent endocarditis, no operative deaths, and only one late death. Muehrcke reported the Cleveland Clinic experiences of MVrep for bacterial endocarditis in 1997.[2] Between 1985 and 1995, 102 of 146 patients (70%) underwent MVrep for mitral IE. Every effort was made to avoid implanting any foreign material in patients with active endocarditis. In patients with acute endocarditis, prosthetic ring annuloplasty was performed in 38% of cases. They concluded that MVrep results

in reduced hospital mortality and improved long-term survival. Lee and colleagues[9] reported 71 consecutive patients who underwent surgery for mitral IE. Endocarditis was divided into 3 stages: uncontrolled and active (n = 24), partially treated (n = 17), and healed (n = 30). The repair rates were 17%, 59%, and 63% for each stage, respectively. The total repair rate was 46%. They concluded that conservative surgery, preferably repair, should be performed, whenever feasible, for mitral IE to maintain left ventricular function. The total number of patients who underwent MVrep for mitral IE in these 4 studies was 197. The repair rate for mitral valve IE ranged between 46% and 80% at these highly experienced centers. The durability of repair was described as acceptable in these reports. However, the benefits of MVrep over MVR in mitral IE cases remained poorly established due to the overall lack of adequately sized and properly designed studies.

Nationwide/"Real World" Cohort Report

Gammie and colleagues reported that 6627 patients underwent mitral valve surgery for mitral IE at 661 Society of Thoracic Surgeons (STS)-participating centers between 1994 and 2003.[11] The repair rate was 29.7% (active IE: 15.9%, treated IE: 40.9%). Although the repair rate for active IE improved from 35.8% to 46.6% during a decade, patients with active IE were less likely to undergo MVrep than those with treated IE. The in-hospital mortality significantly improved in the MVrep group even among the active IE group subjects. The authors supported MVrep, whenever technically feasible, in the setting of mitral IE. Toyoda and colleagues[12] reported real-world outcomes of surgery for native mitral IE. The study population comprised 1970 patients undergoing MVrep (n = 367, 18.6%) and MVR (n = 1603, 81.4%) in the states of New York and California between 1998 and 2010. The repair rates increased from 10.7% to 19.4% over the study period. The propensity-matched cohort included 798 patients: 266 in the MVrep group and 532 in the MVR group. The focus was on the association between mitral reoperation and the surgeon's case volume. MVrep performed for endocarditis by high-volume surgeons was 5 times less likely to require reoperation within 1 year than MVrep performed by low-volume surgeons (<25 cases per year). They concluded that survival rates were better, and the risk of recurrent infections was lower for MVrep than for MVR in active endocarditis patients; MVrep should be the surgery of choice when feasible. Lee and colleagues[13] conducted a nationwide cohort study comparing MVrep and

MVR for mitral IE between January 2000 and December 2013 in Taiwan. During the study period, 1999 patients underwent MV surgery for IE for the first time. The repair rate was 21.2% and the number of patients undergoing MVrep increased during the study period. A total of 352 propensity score–matched patients who underwent MVrep and MVR were eligible for the analysis. They concluded that MVrep for IE showed better perioperative and late outcomes than MVR. However, the beneficial effect of MVrep was not significant in low-volume hospitals.

Operative Techniques

Surgical principles are very important (**Box 1**). Exposure of acute mitral IE reveals leaflet perforations, vegetations of various sizes, and extension (**Fig. 1**). Owing to the possibility of recurrent infection in MVrep for mitral IE due to incomplete resection of the infected valvular tissue, all macroscopically involved tissues are largely resected without any concern for the possibility of repair. The surgical steps are listed in **Box 1**. The first step involves wide resection of the infected sites of the valve, including a strip of at least 2 mm of normal valvular tissue as described by Dreyfus.[1] The infected fragile chordae are also resected. The intact marginal chordae should be carefully preserved. The mitral annular abscess is examined along the posterior annulus. Reparative procedures for mitral IE have not changed significantly from those described in the series of Dreyfus in 1990, except chordal reconstruction with expanded polytetrafluoroethylene (ePTFE) sutures. In case of a mitral annular abscess, the abscess is opened and aggressively debrided, and the defect is corrected using a properly tailored autologous pericardial patch. The presence of a mitral annular abscess does not automatically imply valve replacement; annulus reconstruction must be required for performing either MVrep or MVR. After resecting a small area of infection of the posterior leaflet, placing a direct suture may be possible. In case of anterior leaflet perforation and commissure area infection, especially in the presence of acute infection, treated or untreated autologous pericardium may be used as a patch graft because of the fragility of the remaining leaflet tissue, which may be prone to tearing after a direct suture is placed (**Figs. 2 and 3**).

The key factors determining reparability are the extent and location of tissue destruction by the endocarditic process and the quality of the remaining tissue after radical resection of the infected tissue. Shang and colleagues suggested that MVrep should not be attempted when more than 50% to 60% of the posterior leaflet is absent or when more than 10% to 20% of the free edge of the anterior leaflet has been destroyed.[14] Similar to Dreyfus's observation in 1990, Shang and colleagues also noted that considerable destruction of the anterior leaflet did not necessarily mandate replacement because an autologous pericardial patch could reconstruct a large percentage of the body of the anterior leaflet. Defauw and colleagues reported that two-thirds of the free edge of the mitral valve and one commissure must be intact in order to attempt repair.[15] The repair rate in their study was 66% (of 149 patients) between 2000 and 2017.

Late results of pericardial patch grafting for anterior leaflet perforation indicate it to be a reliable procedure.[10,16–18] A relatively large autologous pericardial patch graft is sutured along the remnants of the anterior and posterior leaflets, resembling the sail of a yacht during systole. By placing the magic stitches at the commissure area, chordal reconstruction using ePTFE sutures is performed along the unsupported autologous pericardium at the anterior leaflet to achieve good coaptation of the anterior and posterior parts of the autologous pericardium (**Fig. 4**, Video 1). Chordal transfer from the posterior leaflet (flip-over technique) may also be effective. Chordal reconstruction using ePTFE sutures is a feasible technique for correcting the prolapse of the remnant leaflet. The combination of chordal

---

Box 1
Surgical steps of mitral valve repair for infective endocarditis

Step 1. Radical resection of infected tissue

Leaflet, chordae, annular abscess debridement

Step 2. Annulus reconstruction using pericardium (if required)

Step 3. Decision-making whether remaining leaflet tissue is sufficient (two-thirds free margin of AML/PML and one commissure: intact)

Step 4. Restore leaflet deficit using pericardium

Step 5. Chordal reconstruction by chordal transfer/ePTFE sutures

Step 6. Ring annuloplasty in the case of annular dilatation

Step 7. Assessment of mitral valve repair by intraoperative TEE

Abbreviations: AML/PML, anterior posterior mitral leaflet; ePTFE, expanded polytetrafluoroethylene; TEE, transesophageal echocardiography.

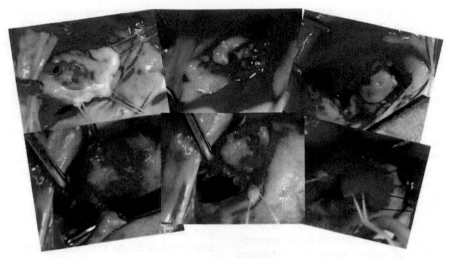

Fig. 1. Operative findings of mitral valve infective endocarditis.

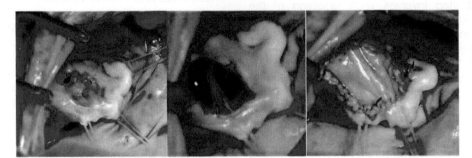

Fig. 2. Perforations of anterior mitral leaflet and patch closure using autologous pericardium.

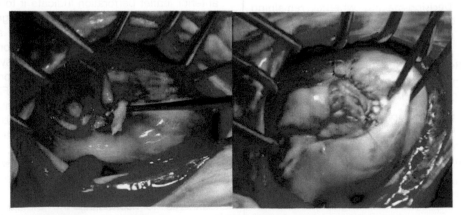

Fig. 3. Infective endocarditis at commissure area and repair using autologous pericardium.

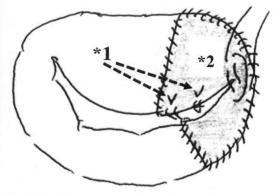

Fig. 4. Leaflet reconstruction using autologous pericardium and ePTFE suture (*1: chordal reconstruction using ePTFE. *2: magic stitch to make a good coaptation).

reconstruction and anterior leaflet patching is a complex procedure and requires an experienced surgeon. Redundancy of the autologous pericardium at the anterior leaflet is mandatory. In such cases, a prosthetic ring is required to create a good coaptation area.

To reduce the chances of early redo surgery for residual or recurrent mitral regurgitation (MR), immediate assessment of this complex MVrep using intraoperative transesophageal echocardiography is mandatory. In our practice, a second pump run is always indicated in cases of residual MR of the mild grade or more. The second pump run incidence was 8.8%, and rerepair was accomplished in all our cases.[19] Freedom from reoperation at 5 years was 90% in active mitral IE and 99% in healed mitral IE cases.

Reports from a Single Institute (2000–2020)

The number of patients who underwent MVrep for mitral IE ranged from 34 to 155 (**Table 1**). The case volumes in each institution during an average of 14 years are quite limited. The repair rate varied from 33% to 86% based on the surgeon's discretion. Iung and colleagues reported that the surgical techniques used in their study were highly specialized and could not be widely extrapolated.[20] The procedures included leaflet resection, transposition of chordae, chordal shortening, pericardial patch repair, partial homograft insertion, and prosthetic ring annuloplasty. However, they reported that the good results obtained using MVrep should lead to its diffusion, as has previously been the case with degenerative causes. Ruttmann and colleagues compared the surgical results between MVrep (n = 34) and MVR (n = 34) for mitral IE without performing randomization.[21] They used leaflet reconstruction with treated autologous pericardium, annular reconstruction with autologous pericardium, chordal transposition, rotation paracommissural sliding plasty, and ring annuloplasty. They observed that asking a surgeon to perform a procedure that he or she is not convinced about or lacks a high level of experience in may be unethical. Therefore, randomized trials are unlikely to be feasible regarding the choice of these 2 surgical techniques. They concluded that MVrep offers excellent early and late results in terms of event-free survival after surgery. Doukas and colleagues reported the use of MVrep (n = 36) for active culture-positive mitral IE.[22] They concluded that MVrep for active mitral IE was associated with low operative mortality and provided satisfactory freedom from recurrent infections and repeat

Table 1
Reports of mitral valve repair for mitral infective endocarditis (2000–2020)

Study (Year)	No of Repair	(Acute/ Healed)	Repair Rate (%)	Mean Age	Hsp Mortality (%)	Survival
Iung et al,[20] 2004	63	(25/38)	81	50 ± 17	3.2	93 + 4% (7 y)
Ruttmann et al,[21] 2005	34	(34/-)	50	52 ± 17	11.8	85% (5 y)
Doukas et al,[22] 2006	36	(36/-)	46	53	2.8	93% (5 y)
Shang et al,[14] 2009	56	(36/20)	63	48	5.3	91% (5 y)
Shimokawa et al,[23] 2009	78	(14/64)	86	50 ± 15	0	90 ± 5% (10 y)
Jung et al,[24] 2011	41	(41/-)	40	34 ± 17	0	98% (5 y)
Perrotta et al,[25] 2018	76	(NA)	54	60	1	77 ± 6% (10 y)
Tepsuwan et al,[26] 2019	38	(38/-)	33	44 ± 16	2.6	72% (10 y)
Solari et al,[27] 2019	155	(155/-)	81	60 ± 14	11.6	65 ± 5% (10 y)
Defauw et al,[15] 2020	97	(NA)	66	57 ± 13	12.4	66.5% (10 y)
Okada et al,[19] 2020	147	(49/98)	86	50 ± 18	0.7	89 ± 4% (10 y)

operations as well as improved survival. Shang and colleagues reported early surgical therapy and the aggressive use of repair for mitral IE.[14] They also concluded that MVrep for mitral IE offered a long-term survival advantage over MVR. Shimokawa and colleagues reported 78 cases of MVrep for mitral IE (active n = 14, healed n = 64).[23] They observed that MVrep for mitral IE was associated with low operative mortality and morbidity, and its long-term durability was comparable to that of repair for degenerative MR. Jung and colleagues analyzed MVrep (n = 41) and MVR (n = 61) for active mitral IE without performing randomization[24] and found no significant difference in the long-term survival and event-free survival between the 2 groups. Perrotta and Tepsuwan reported that MVrep for mitral IE is associated with excellent midterm and long-term results in selected patients.[25,26] Solari and colleagues described the use of repair-oriented surgery for active mitral IE.[27] They applied a wide armamentarium of repair techniques including autologous pericardium repair, tricuspid autograft, and mitral homograft as a leaflet. Early surgery and repair-oriented surgery for mitral IE were recommended. Solari and colleagues compared the clinical results of MVrep with patch and MVrep without patch. They concluded that patients could benefit from complex MVrep even if patch material was necessary for valve repair. We used treated autologous pericardium as a leaflet substrate, ePTFE sutures (CV-5) for chordal reconstruction, and a prosthetic ring if required.[19] Our basic concept in mitral IE repair involves radical resection of the infected tissue and functional reconstruction of the mitral valve without residual MR. We do not hesitate to use a second pump run to minimize residual MR after MVrep for mitral IE. In these 11 reports, freedom from redo surgery for recurrent MR rates or reinfection after MVrep rates ranged from very high to acceptable.

DISCUSSION

This review found that MVrep, using a wide armamentarium of reparative procedures, has the potential to improve late outcomes in patients undergoing mitral valve surgery for mitral IE. Early repair-oriented surgery is recommended for mitral IE to prevent worsening heart failure and continuing valve destruction due to the infection.

The advantages of MVrep over replacement are well established in terms of preservation of left ventricular function, low perioperative mortality, and freedom from valve-related events after surgery for severe degenerative MR. However, no randomized clinical trials comparing MVrep and MVR have

been conducted, even among patients with degenerative MR. The accumulation of retrospective observational studies and spread of knowledge of repair techniques at academic conferences have gained the attitude of the heart valve team.

The single-institutional series on MVrep for mitral IE in the 1990s by Carpentier's group and the Cleveland Clinic Foundation stimulated us to consider the possibility of MVrep for mitral IE to obtain better surgical results. Early in the 1990s, Prof. Carpentier taught me that the surgeon should try to repair the affected valve in mitral IE soon after identification of the organism before the destruction of the mitral apparatus occurs. Our initial experience of successful repairs for mitral IE in terms of postoperative care and freedom from valve-related events had a great impact on our team members. Our experience with treated autologous pericardium in MVrep for rheumatic MR since 1991 has been very helpful in valve repair for mitral IE cases.[17]

Dreyfus noted that the only limiting factor in MVrep is the extent of the lesions. Although he reported that determining whether enough mitral valve tissue was available after radical resection of the infected tissue was easy, the reparability rates differ depending on the surgeon's skill and experience. The intactness of two-thirds of the free edge of the mitral valve and of one commissure is the anatomic criterion by Defauw and colleagues that is generally accepted.[15] After radical resection of the infected tissue, the leaflet tissue deficit is restored using treated or fresh autologous pericardium. Extension of the leaflet using treated or fresh autologous pericardium is not a challenging procedure but rather a standard procedure to increase the good coaptation area in patients with insufficient leaflet tissue.[10,17] Autologous pericardium is a good substrate to expand the reparability in complex mitral valve disease, including mitral valve IE.

Chordal reconstruction involves chordal transfer or using ePTFE sutures to create a competent valve. Although surgeons still hesitate to use prosthetic materials such as prosthetic rings and ePTFE sutures for chordal reconstruction in patients with early-stage active mitral IE, reinfection rates are very low after implantation of prosthetic materials. A wide armamentarium of repair techniques is available even in the setting of active mitral IE.

As the number of patients who require surgical treatment of mitral IE is very limited, systemic reviews and meta-analyses have attempted to compare the clinical results of MVrep and MVR in the setting of mitral IE. Feringa and colleagues compared the clinical outcomes of MVrep (n = 470) and MVR (n = 724) based on 24 studies published between January 1980 and May 2005.[3] They concluded that MVrep is associated with good clinical in-hospital and long-term results among patients undergoing surgery for mitral IE. Harkey and colleagues also analyzed MVrep (n = 2906) and MVR (n = 6072) based on 14 studies published between 1997 and 2014.[4] They demonstrated that MVrep was associated with better clinical results than MVR in terms of freedom from reoperation, reinfection, and midterm mortality. The repaired mitral valve is durable and resistant to infection in the setting of either acute or healed endocarditis. According to the reports of experienced centers, MVrep for mitral IE demonstrated improved event-free survival.

Byrne and colleagues reported the STS Clinical Practice Guideline for surgical management of endocarditis.[5] If the infectious disease is limited to the valvular tissue, MVrep is the preferred surgical option based on the evidence of single-institution reports published between 2004 and 2007.[20–22,28,29] They reported the advantages of MVrep over MVR, such as better preservation of left ventricular function and a reduced rate of prosthetic valve-related complications. The current American Association for Thoracic Surgery and European Society of Cardiology/European Association for Cardio-Thoracic Surgery (ESC/EACTS) guidelines also recommend valve repair whenever possible, particularly when IE affects the mitral valve without causing significant destruction. The ESC/EACTS guidelines state that intraoperative assessment of the valve after debridement is of paramount importance to evaluate whether the remaining tissue is of sufficient quality to achieve a durable repair. The need for a patch to achieve a competent valve is not associated with worse results in terms of recurrence of IE or MR when performed by experienced surgeons. Successful MVrep can be achieved in up to 80% of patients by experienced teams, but such results may not be duplicated in nonspecialist centers.

Bolling commented on the marked variability in the frequency of MVrep, and the median number of mitral valve surgeries per year was 5 (range, 1–166), according to the STS database.[30] One of the characteristics that decreased the repair rate was the presence of active endocarditis. Stahel and colleagues analyzed the role of the surgeon's experience in predicting the probability of a successful MVrep.[31] They pointed out that a preoperative assessment of 7 variables including endocarditis can accurately predict the risk of MVrep failure. As Antunes noted, it is widely accepted that MVrep, whenever possible, yields better short-term and long-term results than replacement, even for infected native valves.[32,33]

Surgeons should therefore become acquainted with and master the multiple techniques that have proved useful in this setting. The solution to realizing the potential of MVrep in IE may be education and exposure.

SUMMARY

MVrep, using a wide armamentarium of reparative procedures, has the potential to improve late outcomes in patients undergoing mitral valve surgery for mitral IE. Early repair-oriented surgery is recommended for mitral IE.

CLINICS CARE POINTS

- Guidelines currently recommend MVrep whenever possible for patients with mitral IE in terms of short- and long-term clinical results.

- In general, two-thirds free edge of mitral valve and one commissure need to remain intact in order to attempt repair.

- MVrep using a wide armamentarium of reparative procedures including autologous pericardium as a leaflet substitute, ePTFE for chordal reconstruction, and a prosthetic ring has a possibility to expand reparability of mitral IE.

- Intraoperative transesophageal echocardiography is mandatory to assess immediate operative results to reduce early redo operation for this kind of complex repair.

DISCLOSURE

None.

SUPPLEMENTARY DATA

Supplementary data related to this article can be found online at https://doi.org/10.1016/j.ccl.2021.01.005.

REFERENCES

1. Dreyfus G, Serraf A, Jebara VA, et al. Valve repair in acute endocarditis. Ann Thorac Surg 1990;49:706–13.
2. Muehrcke DD, Cosgrove DM 3rd, Lytle BW, et al. Is there an advantage to repairing infected mitral valves? Ann Thorac Surg 1997;63:1718–24.
3. Feringa HHH, Shaw LJ, Poldermans D, et al. Mitral valve repair and replacement in endocarditis: a

systemic review of literature. Ann Thorac Surg 2007; 83:564–71.

4. Harky A, Hof A, Garner M, et al. Mitral valve repair or replacement in native valve endocarditis? systemic review and meta-analysis. J Card Surg 2018;33:364–71.

5. Byrne JG, Rezai K, Sanchez JA, et al. Surgical management of endocarditis: the Society of Thoracic Surgeons clinical practice guideline. Ann Thorac Surg 2011;91:2012–9.

6. AATS Surgical Treatment of Infective Endocarditis Consensus Guidelines Writing Committee Chairs, Pettersson GB, Coselli JS, et al. 2016 the American Association for Thoracic Surgery (AATS) consensus guidelines: surgical treatment of infective endocarditis: executive summary. J Thorac Cardiovasc Surg 2017;153:1241–58.e29.

7. Habib G, Lancellotti P, Antunes MJ, et al. 2015 ESC guidelines for the management of infective endocarditis: the Task Force for the management of infective endocarditis of the European Society of Cardiology (ESC). Endorsed by: European association for Cardio-Thoracic surgery (EACTS), the European association of Nuclear Medicine (EANM). Eur Heart J 2015;36:3075–128.

8. Pagani FD, Monaghan HL, Deeb GM, et al. Mitral valve reconstruction for active and healed endocarditis. Circulation 1996;94(9 Suppl):II133–8.

9. Lee EM, Shapiro LM, Wells FC. Conservative operation for infective endocarditis of the mitral valve. Ann Thorac Surg 1998;65:1087–92.

10. Chauvaud S, Jebara V, Chachques JC, et al. Valve extension with glutaraldehyde-preserved autologous pericardium. Results in mitral valve repair. J Thorac Cardiovasc Surg 1991;102:171–8.

11. Gammie JS, O'Brien SM, Griffith BP, et al. Surgical treatment of mitral valve endocarditis in North America. Ann Thorac Surg 2005;80:2199–204.

12. Toyoda N, Itagaki S, Egorova NN, et al. Real-world outcomes of surgery for native mitral valve endocarditis. J Thorac Cardiovasc Surg 2017;154:1906–12.e9.

13. Lee HA, Cheng YT, Wu VC, et al. Nationwide cohort study of mitral valve repair versus replacement for infective endocarditis. J Thorac Cardiovasc Surg 2018;156:1473–83.e2.

14. Shang E, Forrest GN, Chizmar T, et al. Mitral valve infective endocarditis: benefit of early operation and aggressive use of repair. Ann Thorac Surg 2009;87:1728–34.

15. Defauw RJ, Tomšič A, van Brakel TJ, et al. A structured approach to native mitral valve infective endocarditis: is repair better than replacement? Eur J Cardiothorac Surg 2020;58:544–50.

16. Sareyyupoglu B, Schaff HV, Suri RM, et al. Safety and durability of mitral valve repair for anterior leaflet perforation. J Thorac Cardiovasc Surg 2010;139:1488–93.

17. Shomura Y, Okada Y, Nasu M, et al. Late results of mitral valve repair with glutaraldehyde-treated autologous pericardium. Ann Thorac Surg 2013;95:2000–5.

18. Quinn RW, Wang L, Foster N, et al. Long-term performance of fresh autologous pericardium for mitral valve leaflet repair. Ann Thorac Surg 2020;109:36–41.

19. Okada Y, Nakai T, Muro T, et al. Mitral valve repair for infective endocarditis: Kobe experience. Asian Cardiovasc Thorac Ann 2020;28:384–9.

20. Iung B, Rousseau-Paziaud J, Cormier B, et al. Contemporary results of mitral valve repair for infective endocarditis. J Am Coll Cardiol 2004;43:386–92.

21. Ruttmann E, Legit C, Poelzl G, et al. Mitral valve repair provides improved outcome over replacement in active infective endocarditis. J Thorac Cardiovasc Surg 2005;130:765–71.

22. Doukas G, Oc M, Alexiou C, et al. Mitral valve repair for active culture positive infective endocarditis. Heart 2006;92:361–3.

23. Shimokawa T, Kasegawa H, Matsuyama S, et al. Long-term outcome of mitral valve repair for infective endocarditis. Ann Thorac Surg 2009;88:733–9.

24. Jung SH, Je HG, Choo SJ, et al. Surgical results of active infective native mitral valve endocarditis: repair versus replacement. Eur J Cardiothorac Surg 2011;40:834–9.

25. Perrotta S, Fröjd V, Lepore V, et al. Surgical treatment for isolated mitral valve endocarditis: a 16-year single-centre experience. Eur J Cardiothorac Surg 2018;53:576–81.

26. Tepsuwan T, Rimsukcharoenchai C, Tantraworasin A, et al. Comparison between mitral valve repair and replacement in active infective endocarditis. Gen Thorac Cardiovasc Surg 2019;67:1030–7.

27. Solari S, De Kerchove L, Tamer S, et al. Active infective mitral valve endocarditis: is a repair-oriented surgery safe and durable? Eur J Cardiothorac Surg 2019;55:256–62.

28. de Kerchove L, Vanoverschelde JL, Poncelet A, et al. Reconstructive surgery in active mitral valve endocarditis: feasibility, safety and durability. Eur J Cardiothorac Surg 2007;31:592–9.

29. Feringa HHH, Bax JJ, Klein P, et al. Outcome after mitral valve repair for acute and healed infective endocarditis. Eur J Cardiothorac Surg 2006;29:367–73.

30. Bolling SF, Li S, O'Brien SM, et al. Predictors of mitral valve repair: clinical and surgeon factors. Ann Thorac Surg 2010;90:1904–12.

31. Stahel HTT, Kammermann A, Gahl B, et al. A simple preoperative score including the surgeon's experience to predict the probability of a successful mitral valve repair. Interact Cardiovasc Thorac Surg 2017;24:841–7.

32. Antunes MJ. Mitral valve repair versus replacement for infective endocarditis. What is better in the "real world"? J Thorac Cardiovasc Surg 2018;156:1471–2.

33. Antunes MJ. Mitral valve repair versus replacement for infective endocarditis, again. J Thorac Cardiovasc Surg 2018;158:e33.

Optimal Timing of Surgery for Patients with Active Infective Endocarditis

Takeshi Kitai, MD, PhD[a],*, Akiko Masumoto, MD[a], Taiji Okada, MD, PhD[a],
Tadaaki Koyama, MD, PhD[b], Yutaka Furukawa, MD, PhD[a]

KEYWORDS

- Infective endocarditis • Surgery • Complication • Stroke

KEY POINTS

- As delays in diagnosis and initiation of therapy could lead to worse outcomes in patients with infective endocarditis (IE), identification of indication for surgical intervention and its optimal timing are crucial.
- Indications for surgery are based on cardiac and extracardiac complications.
- One of the most common clinical dilemmas regarding surgical intervention for IE is optimal timing of surgery for patients with concomitant neurologic complications such as stroke, intracranial hemorrhage, and mycotic aneurysm.
- Once IE is diagnosed or even suspected, 4 sets of examinations, including transthoracic echocardiography, transesophageal echocardiography, contrast-enhanced computed tomography, and cerebral MRI should be performed to comprehensively assess the necessity of further management, including surgery.

INTRODUCTION

Infective endocarditis (IE) is a rare but serious condition with a dismal prognosis. The incidence of IE has increased over the past few decades to 3 to 10 cases per 100,000 people annually.[1–4] The highest incidence is observed among persons aged 70 to 80 years, with a twofold to threefold higher male predominance. It should be noted that almost half of IE cases occur in individuals without a diagnosed structural disease of the heart.[1] Despite improvements in diagnostic modalities and therapeutic methods, including antibiotic therapy and surgical techniques, IE still poses a clinical challenge to both diagnosis and management and leads to a high mortality rate. The in-hospital mortality rate was reported to be 18% to 25%, with the 1-year mortality rate reaching up to 40%.[5–14] A recent study indicated that the mortality rate for IE was 2.4 per 100,000 people in the United States.[15]

The keys to improving outcomes include an early diagnosis of definite IE, a prompt identification of high-risk patients who have intracardiac and extracardiac complications, and appropriate management, including surgery for high-risk patients. Delays in diagnosis and initiation of therapy lead to complications and worse clinical outcomes.[16] The main complications of IE are embolic events and subsequent bleeding, persistent bacteremia, and heart failure mainly

Funding: None.
Conflicts of interest: None.
[a] Department of Cardiovascular Medicine, Kobe City Medical Center General Hospital, 2-1-1 Minatojima-minamimachi, Chuo-ku, Kobe 6500047, Japan; [b] Department of Cardiovascular Surgery, Kobe City Medical Center General Hospital, 2-1-1 Minatojima-minamimachi, Chuo-ku, Kobe 6500047, Japan
* Corresponding author.
E-mail address: t-kitai@kcho.jp

because of valvular regurgitation. Historically, there have been controversies surrounding the optimal indication and timing for surgery, especially for patients presenting with neurologic complications.

This article reviews the necessary workup for patients with suspected IE and proposes a state-of-art patient flow chart to guide subsequent clinical management, focusing on surgical indications (**Fig. 1**). When indications for surgery arise after evaluation proposed by the algorithm *and* the patients present with concomitant neurologic complications, an additional evaluation process is necessary before arrangements for surgery are made (**Fig. 2**).

INITIAL ASSESSMENT AND DIAGNOSIS OF INFECTIVE ENDOCARDITIS

IE develops from underlying valvular or nonvalvular cardiac structural abnormalities and results in blood flow turbulence and disruption of the endocardial endothelium. Subsequently, platelet aggregation and fibrin disposition are induced to the damaged endothelium, causing lesions defined as nonbacterial thrombotic endocarditis, which serve as a foundation for adhesion by circulating bacteria or fungi in the bloodstream.[17–19] The lesions predominantly involve the valves, but also can involve the mural endocardium.[20,21] Besides the infection damaging the valve, there is also a risk of embolization and stroke.

Diagnosis of IE is difficult and is often delayed until serious infection or complications are evident.[22–24] The modified Duke criteria are the most commonly used and validated criteria for IE diagnosis and classification.[25] However, considering the vast heterogeneity of clinical presentations of IE, the modified Duke criteria should be used in combination with circumspect clinical judgment. Two major components of the Duke

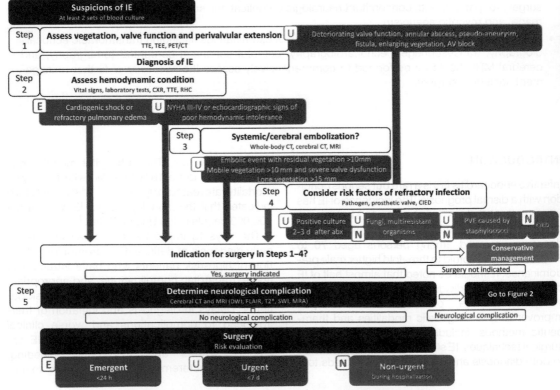

Fig. 1. State-of-the-art patient algorithm for evaluation of suspected IE. After the initial assessment of vegetation, valve function, and perivalvular extension in step 1, the evaluations in steps 2 to 4 are conducted to seek indications for surgery. Special consideration should be given to PVE and cardiac device infection (CDI). When indications for surgery arise after evaluations in steps 1 to 4, and the patient presents with concomitant neurologic complications, the evaluations in step 5 are added (see **Fig. 2**) before surgery. Before surgery, surgical risk should be considered and weighed against the benefits of avoiding further complications with early surgery. Abx, antibiotics; AV block, atrioventricular block; CIED, cardiac implantable electronic device; CXR, chest radiograph; DWI, diffusion-weighted imaging; E, emergent surgery within 24 hours; FLAIR, fluid-attenuated inversion recovery; Lac, lactate; N, nonurgent surgery or elective surgery during hospitalization; RHC, right heart catheterization; sBP, systolic blood pressure; SWI, susceptibility-weighted imaging; U, urgent surgery within 7 days.

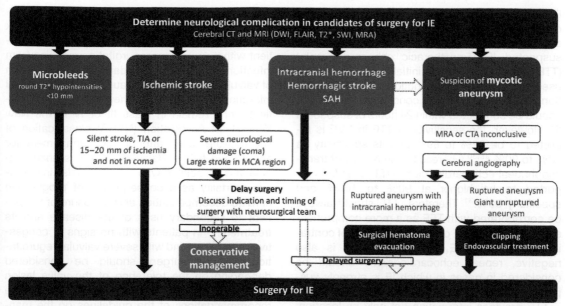

Fig. 2. Indications for surgery in patients with neurologic complications. When indications for surgery arise *and* concomitant neurologic complications are detected on cerebral CT and/or cerebral MRI, each neurologic complication should be evaluated and managed to determine if cardiac surgery is feasible. DWI, diffusion-weighted imaging; FLAIR, fluid-attenuated inversion recovery; MCA, middle cerebral artery; SAH, subarachnoid hemorrhage; SWI, susceptibility-weighted imaging; TIA, transient ischemic attack.

criteria include the results from blood culture and echocardiography.

Positive Blood Culture and Culture-Negative Endocarditis

In addition to the diagnostic purposes, results from blood culture are also crucial for determining appropriate antibiotic therapy, which is the mainstay in the management of IE. Antibiotic therapy should be initiated promptly and targeted to the organism isolated from the blood cultures with a prolonged duration regardless of the timing of surgery. Although *Streptococcus viridans* was the most commonly identified pathogen in the 1960s, the epidemiologic profile of IE has changed recently, with *Staphylococcus aureus* being the predominant causative organism.[20] Causative organisms are associated with the development of both intracardiac and extracardiac complications. *S aureus* is reported to be associated with more frequent stroke, systemic emboli, and persistent bacteremia.[26] A recent study using propensity-matched analysis including more than 700 patients with *S aureus* left-sided native valve endocarditis (NVE) showed that intracardiac abscess and left ventricular ejection fraction less than 40% were independent predictors of in-hospital mortality, whereas intracardiac abscess and valve perforation were independent predictors of 1-year mortality.[27] Moreover, the characteristics of the patients

have also evolved, with a trend toward increased age, more frequent presence of prosthetic valve endocarditis (PVE), and higher frequency of cardiac implantable electric device (CIED) infection, which result in the increasing severity of the patient's condition. Accordingly, antibiotic therapy alone is sometimes insufficient for these high-risk patients, and the number of surgeries performed for IE has been increasing.[28]

Although the diagnosis of IE is contingent on positive blood cultures, 5% to 10% of infections are found to be culture negative. This condition, known as culture-negative endocarditis, is very challenging in terms of the selection of antibiotic therapy. Fastidious bacterial organisms, including fungi or nonbacterial pathogens, can cause culture-negative endocarditis; however, most cases of culture-negative endocarditis in clinical practice are often caused by prior administration of antibiotics before blood culture collection. The condition of negative or unknown causative organisms can influence the indication of surgery. Withdrawal of antibiotics and repeated blood cultures until an organism is isolated might be a consideration to improve diagnosis.

Role of a Complete Echocardiographic Evaluation

Another important component of the modified Duke criteria is the echocardiographic evaluation.

Echocardiography is an important tool for the diagnosis of IE, and is recommended as an initial and essential imaging modality in all patients with suspected IE. Transthoracic echocardiography (TTE), which is often the initial study, should be used to assess valve dysfunction, ventricular function, and hemodynamic conditions. Initial TTE should be conducted within 24 hours of suspected IE. However, the sensitivity of TTE in NVE is reported to be 82% to 89% and its specificity as 70% to 90%,[29,30] whereas the sensitivity of transesophageal echocardiography (TEE) in NVE is reported to be higher at 90% to 100% and specificity 90%.[31] Therefore, TTE should always be corroborated with TEE as a more comprehensive evaluation for IE only in the absence of contraindications for TEE. Even when TEE is also negative, repeat echocardiography should be considered in cases in which IE is strongly suspected based on clinical judgment.[32,33]

TTE provides information not only on location, size, and mobility of vegetation, but also on the indication of the development of more extensive complications such as annular abscess, pseudoaneurysm, fistula formation, and disruption of the integrity of native or prosthetic valves. However, TTE is not suitable for the detection of small vegetations or for evaluations on prosthetic valves, and it may be technically inadequate in the presence of lung disease or body habitus.[34]

Conversely, TEE has higher sensitivity than TTE and is better suited for the detection of cardiac complications with sensitivity, specificity, and positive and negative predictive values of 87%, 95%, and 91% and 92%, respectively.[34] Therefore, TEE is indicated when TTE is positive or nondiagnostic or inconclusive.[35] In one report, TEE resulted in a shift from possible to definite endocarditis in 42% of cases with PVE.[36] Although TEE is essential for the positive or negative diagnosis of IE, the importance of TTE examination as a first step should be noted. The absence of valvular abnormalities or vegetation on TTE has been reported to be associated with a reduced incidence of complications.[37]

Real-time 3-dimensional (3D) TEE adds information on the vegetation morphology and size, and is particularly useful in the assessment of perivalvular extension of the infection, prosthetic valve dehiscence, and valve perforation.[38,39]

ASSESSMENT OF INDICATIONS FOR SURGERY
Hemodynamic Conditions

Among the complications of IE, congestive heart failure has the greatest impact on prognosis. Emergent surgery within 24 hours is indicated regardless of the status of the infection when evidence of pulmonary edema or cardiogenic shock is present. The usual cause of heart failure in a patient with IE is valvular regurgitation resulting from infection-induced valvular damage. Embolization of valvular vegetation can cause acute myocardial infarction and subsequent heart failure.[40] For patients who remain in class III or IV in the New York Heart Association (NYHA) classification of heart failure, even after initial management for acute heart failure, delayed surgery is unacceptable. It is associated with a dramatic rise in operative mortality as a consequence of progressive cardiac decompensation and exposure of the patient to secondary risks of the disease and its treatment.[41] In patients with no signs of congestive heart failure and with severe valvular regurgitation, elective surgery should be considered depending on the tolerance of the valve lesion and should be performed in accordance with the recommendations of the guidelines on the management of valvular heart disease.[42–46]

Refractory Infections

Uncontrolled infection encompasses persistent infection, infection due to resistant microorganisms, and locally uncontrolled infection. Persistent infection is arbitrarily defined as fever and persistent positive blood cultures after 7 to 10 days of appropriate antibiotic treatment. In a study of 256 patients with positive blood culture at admission, persistent positive cultures after 48 to 72 hours from the initiation of antibiotic treatment were associated with higher in-hospital mortality.[47] Urgent surgery is warranted to remove the source of infection.

S aureus IE is characterized by an aggressive clinical course associated with severe valvular damage, large vegetation, embolic complications, and overall poor prognosis.[48] Fungal IE, secondary to infection with *Candida* or *Aspergillus*, is often complicated by bulky vegetation, metastatic infection, periannular spread, and embolic events.[49] Surgery is the only means of eradication of infection when IE is caused by multiresistant organisms, including methicillin-resistant *S aureus* and vancomycin-resistant enterococci. Careful microbiological liaison is essential to determine appropriate antibiotic management during the postoperative period.

Cardiac Complications

Cardiac complications of IE are causes of uncontrolled infection associated with increased mortality. Cardiac complications include congestive heart failure caused by valvular damage from the infection, annular abscess, extension of infection into the conduction system leading to atrioventricular blocks, and mycotic aneurysms of the sinus of Valsalva, which can result in pericarditis, hemopericardium, cardiac tamponade, or fistulas to the cardiac chambers.[20] Urgent surgery is recommended when cardiac complications are detected to reduce the morbidity and mortality of this disorder.[50–52] Representative cases with cardiac complications requiring surgical interventions are summarized in **Fig. 3**.

In a study including 4681 IE cases, the incidence of fistulous intracardiac complications was 1.6%.[53] The incidence of perivalvular abscess is reported to be 30% to 40%. Perivalvular abscess is associated with a higher mortality and a higher risk of systemic and cerebral embolization.[34,54,55] In addition, perivalvular abscess can extend into adjacent cardiac conduction tissues, leading to atrioventricular block. Involvement of the conduction system by IE is most common in the setting of aortic valve infection, especially vegetation and/or abscess, and is observed between the right and noncoronary cusp, which overlies the intraventricular septum containing the proximal ventricular conduction system. Conversely, perivalvular abscesses should be suspected in the setting of conduction abnormalities in patients with IE.[56] It also should be noted that the aortic valve and annulus are more susceptible to abscess formation and associated complications than the mitral valve and annulus.[34,54,57]

Even if the diagnosis of IE has been achieved, TEE is encouraged to obtain further evaluation of valvular lesions and perivalvular complications. TEE is more sensitive for the detection of myocardial abscesses than TTE.[28] The sensitivity of TEE for the diagnosis of PVE is greater than that of TTE (86%–92% vs 17%–52%, respectively), particularly for assessing mitral valve prosthesis or paravalvular complications.[58–62] However, careful assessment is always required, as even TEE may fail to identify an abscess in difficult imaging situations such as calcification, prosthetic valves, or poor image acquisition. Patients with negative TEE for whom the clinical suspicion for IE is high should undergo repeat TEE 7 to 10 days later.

Systemic Emboli

Prevention and treatment of recurrent or primary embolic events represent a major impetus for surgical intervention in the management of IE.

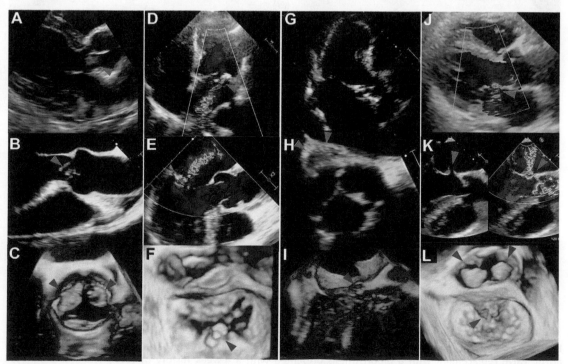

Fig. 3. Representative cases of cardiac complications of IE. (*A–C*) Leaflet aneurysms (*arrowhead*) with perforation in the aortic valves on TTE (*A*), TEE (*B*), and 3D-TEE (*C*). (*D–F*) Leaflet perforation (*arrowhead*) and severe mitral regurgitation in the posterior mitral valve on TTE (*D*), TEE (*E*), and 3D-TEE (*F*). (*G–I*) Periannular abscess (*arrowhead*) in the aortic annuls on TTE (*G*), TEE (*H*), and 3D-TEE (*I*). (*J–L*) Perforation of aorto-mitral curtain (*arrowhead*) and severe mitral regurgitation on TTE (*J*), TEE (*K*), and 3D-TEE (*L*).

Systemic embolism can occur in end organs and/or in soft tissues, including the coronary arteries, kidneys, spleen, liver, lungs, peripheral vasculature, and psoas muscles,[20,63] and may lead to formation of extracardiac abscesses. Embolization has been described in 13% to 44% of patients with IE.[64–66] The known risk factors for embolism are vegetation size, mitral valve involvement, vegetation mobility, and S aureus infection. Vegetation size larger than 10 mm is a predictor of embolic events, and the risk of embolization is particularly high for very large (>15 mm) vegetation.[67,68] Embolism before antimicrobial therapy is a risk factor for new emboli. An increase in vegetation size, despite antimicrobial treatment, may predict subsequent embolic events.[67] The guidelines recommend early surgery if patients experience recurrent embolic events or demonstrate large, mobile vegetation, respectively (Fig. 4).[69] However, the role of vegetation size as the sole indication for surgery has yet to be determined. Similar to the presence of neurologic complications, the incidence of systemic emboli diagnosed by contrast-enhanced computed tomography (CT) is much higher than the incidence diagnosed by symptoms alone. Therefore, contrast-enhanced whole-body CT should be considered in all cases with IE as soon as possible in the absence of contraindications for contrast material. Although antibiotic therapy alone was reported to decrease the incidence of stroke,[70] a recent study showed that early surgical intervention within 48 hours from diagnosis was associated with decreased risk of 6-week embolic

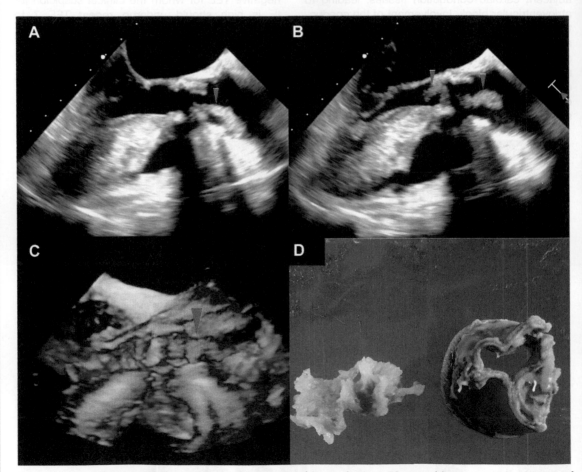

Fig. 4. A case of a large mobile vegetation on the aortic bioprosthesis. A 78-year-old woman with a history of aortic valve replacement with a bioprosthesis presented with a 4-week history of fever, and was diagnosed with PVE. On the mid-esophageal long-axis view, TEE showed a high-echoic 33-mm-long vegetation (*arrowhead*) attached to the prosthesis (A, B). The 3D TEE showed vegetation on the aortic side of the prosthesis (C). The patient underwent urgent resection of the vegetation (D, left) and removal of the infected prosthesis (D, right). The culture obtained from vegetation indicated *Enterococcus faecalis*. The patient was discharged without neurologic deficits after the completion of antibiotic treatment.

events as well as the risk of in-hospital mortality.[71] Furthermore, the incidence of embolic events was reported to be greater with mitral valve vegetation than with aortic valve vegetation. Specifically, the anterior mitral leaflet had the highest risk of embolization.[72,73]

Accordingly, the surgical considerations relative to systemic or neurologic emboli are as follows: (1) surgery is indicated in patients with previous emboli and ongoing high risk of second embolism; (2) surgery is recommended, based on evidence from randomized-controlled trials, in patients at risk of first embolism (vegetation >10 mm in size) when associated with severe valvular regurgitation or stenosis[71]; and (3) surgery may be considered for the primary prevention of embolism in patients without severe valve dysfunction who are considered high risk, such as vegetation greater than 15 mm. Considering that the risk of embolism in left-sided IE is highest during the first week of antibiotics, surgery to prevent embolism must be performed urgently.[67]

Neurologic Complications

IE is complicated by stroke in 20% to 40% of cases, accounting for 65% of embolic events, 90% of which arise in the distribution of the middle cerebral artery (**Fig. 5**).[70] Patients with neurologic complications of IE have been reported to be associated with worse clinical outcomes.[74–77] In transient ischemic attack or silent embolism, surgery is recommended without delay. Although cerebral CT scanning is most often performed, the higher sensitivity of MRI allows for better detection and analysis of cerebral lesions in patients with neurologic symptoms, and this may have a direct impact on the timing of surgery.[78,79] Symptomatic strokes as a complication of IE occur in up to 35% of patients,[66,74,75,80–82] whereas asymptomatic cerebrovascular complications, including ischemic stroke and microhemorrhage may occur in up to 80% of patients.[66,83–85] Therefore, we encourage routine cerebral MRI in all cases with IE with specific sequences, including diffusion-weighted imaging, gradient-recalled fluid-attenuated inversion recovery sequences, T2* sequences, susceptibility-weighted imaging, and magnetic resonance angiography (MRA) with 3D reconstruction to detect mycotic aneurysms. Surgery should not be delayed when indicated, provided that cerebral hemorrhage has been excluded by cranial CT and neurologic damage is not severe.[75]

The most difficult issues surround patients with IE with stroke who require surgery, as there is a risk of hemorrhagic transformation when patients undergo anticoagulation treatment for cardiopulmonary bypass. Patients with intracranial cerebral hemorrhage or complex stroke have significantly higher surgical mortality, and the conventional approach is to defer surgery for at least 4 weeks if indicated in these patients (**Fig. 6**).[75,82] Cerebral microbleeds, defined as hypointense lesions smaller than 10 mm in diameter, seen on T2* or susceptibility-weighted imaging, have been reported to be a risk factor for intracranial cerebral hemorrhage.[86] However, in a study comparing outcomes of surgery performed in 25 (63%) patients with microbleeds and in 24 (71%) patients without microbleeds, there was no significant difference in the de novo stroke incidence postoperatively (16% vs 17%).[87] Although careful monitoring of neurologic deterioration should be performed in patients with microbleeds, its presence is not a contraindication for surgery. **Fig. 1** proposes a state-of-the-art patient flow chart for the evaluation of suspected IE to guide subsequent clinical management, especially for surgical indications, and **Fig. 2** shows an approach for patients with IE with concomitant neurologic complications.

Mycotic aneurysms are uncommon complications of IE that result from septic embolization of vegetation to the arteries, with subsequent spread of infection through the intima and outward through the vessel wall. Mycotic aneurysm can usually develop at points of vessel bifurcation,[88] and are often detected with angiography, and/or CT and MRA with 3D reconstructions (**Fig. 7**). The overall mortality rate among patients with IE with mycotic aneurysms is as high as 60%. Because mycotic aneurysm can rupture and cause intracranial hemorrhage and sudden death,[20,24] it should be treated immediately and appropriately. Early cardiac surgery may be considered in patients with cerebral bleeding from an isolated mycotic aneurysm, in whom neurosurgical or endovascular intervention may produce a sufficient reduction in the risk of recurrent bleeding to permit cardiopulmonary bypass.[89,90]

TIMELY INDICATION AND RISK EVALUATION OF SURGERY

The goal of surgery is resection and debridement of infected tissue, reconstruction of cardiac structures, and removal of the source of embolism. When indications for surgery arise after evaluations in steps 1 to 4 of the algorithm (see **Fig. 1**), and there are no neurologic complications, surgery should be arranged in a timely manner. When there is an indication for surgery *and* concomitant neurologic complications, additional

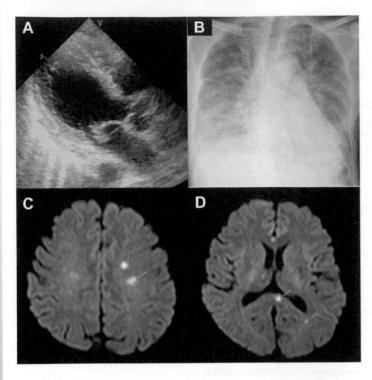

Fig. 5. A case of mitral valve endocarditis complicated with multiple embolic stroke. A 57-year-old man with atopic dermatitis presented with a 3-day history of fever and malaise. Blood culture was positive for methicillin-susceptible *S aureus*, and he presented plantar petechiae. Transthoracic echocardiography revealed highly mobile vegetation (*arrowhead*) attached to the anterior leaflet of the mitral valve and severe mitral regurgitation (*A*). The patient developed acute pulmonary edema on the third day of admission. Chest radiography showed bilateral congestion (*B*). Cerebral MRI showed multiple bihemispheric acute ischemic lesions as hyper-intensity signals (*arrowhead*) in diffusion-weighted image sequences (*C, D*). The patient underwent emergent mitral valve replacement and developed no further neurologic complications after surgery.

assessment should be performed (see **Fig. 2**), and surgery should be planned if surgical risks are acceptable compared with the benefits of surgery.

Ironically, the presence of cardiac and extracardiac complications indicating surgery adds to the surgical risk for active IE, as these conditions

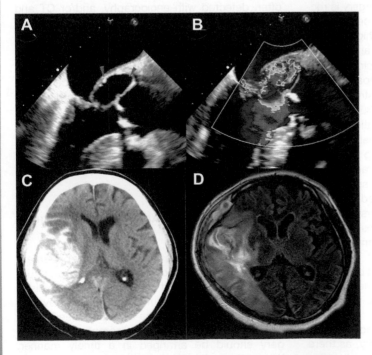

Fig. 6. A case of bicuspid aortic valve endocarditis with large hemorrhagic stroke. A 72-year-old man who was initially treated with antibiotics for Group B streptococcal bacteremia in another institution developed dysarthria and left-sided hemiparesis. Emergent cerebral angiography showed occlusion of the right M2 segment, where thrombus was successfully retrieved. TTE showed vegetation attached to the leaflet of the bicuspid aortic valve and perforation (*arrowhead*) of the aorto-mitral curtain (*A*). TEE revealed severe regurgitation from the sinus of Valsalva to the left atrium (*B*). The patient experienced coma 3 days after the angiography. Cerebral CT images showed hemorrhagic transformation of large lobar infarctions in the right middle cerebral artery region (*C*). Cerebral MRI showed bleeding in fluid-attenuated inversion recovery sequences (*D*). A decompressive craniotomy was conducted, but the patient remained unconscious. Because of the large hemorrhagic infarction and coma, cardiac surgery was deemed unfeasible. Conservative therapy with antibiotics was resumed, and the patient died of respiratory failure 1 month later.

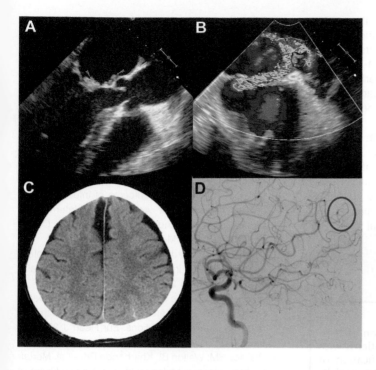

Fig. 7. A case of mitral valve endocarditis complicated with subarachnoid hemorrhage and mycotic aneurysm. A 59-year-old man with known mitral valve P3 prolapse presented with a 3-day history of fever and finger agnosia. TEE showed mobile vegetation (*arrowhead*) attached to the jet lesion of the mitral regurgitant flow (*A*). Severe mitral regurgitation was observed on TEE (*B*). Based on these findings, urgent cardiac surgery was warranted to prevent further embolization; however, subarachnoid hemorrhage was observed in the left occipital lobe with cerebral CT (*C*). Therefore, double-subtraction angiography (DSA) was planned. DSA of the left internal carotid artery showed 2 mycotic aneurysms each at the end of the left angular artery (*circle*) and in the left anterior cerebral artery A2 portion (*D*). The patient was scheduled for embolization of the mycotic aneurysm using N-butyl 2-cyanoacrylate before the cardiac surgery. On day following the embolization, the patient underwent resection of vegetation and mitral valve repair without any additional complications.

deteriorate hemodynamic status and organ dysfunction. Ultimately, the perceived risk of the operation determines the threshold for surgery; surgical procedures for active IE present high risk, with an overall in-hospital mortality of 20%. However, merely delaying surgery might lead to possible harm due to the occurrence of additional lethal complications. Thus, one must weigh anticipated surgical risk against the benefits of avoiding further complications with early surgery. When surgery is not indicated, or is indicated and the existing neurologic complications or comorbidities pose too high a risk, conservative therapy with antibiotics is pursued. In the case of a worrisome clinical course, evaluation with TTE and assessments in steps 2 to 4 should be repeated to search for new cardiac and extracardiac complications.

Special Considerations

PVE accounts for 10% to 20% of most cases. In early (within 1 year of surgery) PVE, spread of infection beyond the points of attachment of the valve prosthesis is almost inevitable, and root abscesses and valve dehiscence arise in 60% of cases. Surgical treatment results in improved survival at both immediate and long-term follow-up and a reduced incidence of relapse or need for repeat surgery compared with medical therapy.[91]

When indicated, surgery is best performed urgently, especially when infection is caused by S aureus.[92] In late PVE (after 1 year of surgery), aggressive tissue destruction is less frequent, and early antibiotic therapy can affect a cure in many patients for whom surgery is often unnecessary. An exception is late PVE due to S aureus, for which the prognosis is dismal,[93] thus, urgent surgery is indicated.[94–96]

CIEDs include permanent pacemakers, implantable cardioverter-defibrillators, and cardiac resynchronization therapy devices. CIED infection may involve the generator pocket, device leads, or endocardial surfaces. IE may originate from a pocket infection or occur by seeding of infection to the leads via the bloodstream. Management of CIED infection is difficult, and complete system removal is necessary.[97] Advances in percutaneous techniques have lowered the risk of device extraction.[98]

SUMMARY

We can summarize important keys features for the successful management of IE as follows: (1) prompt and adequate diagnosis of IE itself and initiation of antibiotics; (2) prompt and adequate identification of complications and indications for surgery; and (3) prompt initiation of surgery when faced with surgical risks, especially those with neurologic and hemorrhagic complications. Once IE is diagnosed or even suspected, 4 sets of examinations, including TTE, TEE, contrast-enhanced CT, and cerebral MRI, should be performed to assess the necessity of further management, including surgery, unless there are contraindications for these examinations.

Although robust evidence in the future is required to resolve the controversies regarding the surgical indications for IE, benefits of early surgery have emerged in the past decades. Physicians should promptly assess the patient's conditions and complications with existing modalities in order to recognize the optimal timing for surgery for patients with IE.

CLINICS CARE POINTS

- As delays in diagnosis and initiation of therapy lead to worse outcomes in patients with infective endocarditis (IE), identification of indication for surgical intervention and its optimal timing are crucial.

- Indications for surgery are based on cardiac and extracardiac complications. Once IE is diagnosed, 4 sets of examinations, including transthoracic echocardiography, transesophageal echocardiography, contrast-enhanced computed tomography, and cerebral MRI should be performed.

- One of the most common clinical dilemmas regarding surgical intervention for IE is optimal timing of surgery for patients with concomitant neurologic complications such as stroke, intracranial hemorrhage, and mycotic aneurysm.

ACKNOWLEDGMENTS

None.

REFERENCES

1. Cahill TJ, Prendergast BD. Infective endocarditis. Lancet 2016;387:882–93.
2. Slipczuk L, Codolosa JN, Davila CD, et al. Infective endocarditis epidemiology over five decades: a systematic review. PLoS One 2013;8:e82665.
3. Pant S, Patel NJ, Deshmukh A, et al. Trends in infective endocarditis incidence, microbiology, and valve replacement in the United States from 2000 to 2011. J Am Coll Cardiol 2015;65:2070–6.
4. Bustamante-Munguira J, Mestres CA, Alvarez P, et al. Surgery for acute infective endocarditis: epidemiological data from a Spanish nationwide hospital-based registry. Interact Cardiovasc Thorac Surg 2018;27:498–504.
5. Wang A, Gaca JG, Chu VH. Management considerations in infective endocarditis: a review. JAMA 2018;320:72–83.
6. Cabell CH, Jollis JG, Peterson GE, et al. Changing patient characteristics and the effect on mortality in endocarditis. Arch Intern Med 2002;162:90–4.
7. Murdoch DR, Corey GR, Hoen B, et al. Clinical presentation, etiology, and outcome of infective endocarditis in the 21st century: the International Collaboration on Endocarditis-Prospective Cohort Study. Arch Intern Med 2009;169:463–73.
8. Toyoda N, Chikwe J, Itagaki S, et al. Trends in infective endocarditis in California and New York State, 1998-2013. JAMA 2017;317:1652–60.
9. Thornhill MH, Jones S, Prendergast B, et al. Quantifying infective endocarditis risk in patients with predisposing cardiac conditions. Eur Heart J 2018;39:586–95.
10. Wallace SM, Walton BI, Kharbanda RK, et al. Mortality from infective endocarditis: clinical predictors of outcome. Heart 2002;88:53–60.
11. Chu VH, Cabell CH, Benjamin DK Jr, et al. Early predictors of in-hospital death in infective endocarditis. Circulation 2004;109:1745–9.
12. Hasbun R, Vikram HR, Barakat LA, et al. Complicated left-sided native valve endocarditis in adults: risk classification for mortality. JAMA 2003;289:1933–40.
13. Hill EE, Herijgers P, Claus P, et al. Infective endocarditis: changing epidemiology and predictors of 6-month mortality: a prospective cohort study. Eur Heart J 2007;28:196–203.
14. Wang A, Athan E, Pappas PA, et al. Contemporary clinical profile and outcome of prosthetic valve endocarditis. JAMA 2007;297:1354–61.
15. Roth GA, Dwyer-Lindgren L, Bertozzi-Villa A, et al. Trends and patterns of geographic variation in cardiovascular mortality among US counties, 1980-2014. JAMA 2017;317:1976–92.
16. Cahill TJ, Baddour LM, Habib G, et al. Challenges in infective endocarditis. J Am Coll Cardiol 2017;69:325–44.
17. Holland TL, Baddour LM, Bayer AS, et al. Infective endocarditis. Nat Rev Dis Primers 2016;2:16059.
18. Moreillon P, Que YA. Infective endocarditis. Lancet 2004;363:139–49.
19. Werdan K, Dietz S, Loffler B, et al. Mechanisms of infective endocarditis: pathogen-host interaction and risk states. Nat Rev Cardiol 2014;11:35–50.
20. Mylonakis E, Calderwood SB. Infective endocarditis in adults. N Engl J Med 2001;345:1318–30.
21. AATS Surgical Treatment of Infective Endocarditis Consensus Guidelines Writing Committee Chairs,

Pettersson GB, Coselli JS, et al. 2016 the American Association for Thoracic Surgery (AATS) consensus guidelines: surgical treatment of infective endocarditis: executive summary. J Thorac Cardiovasc Surg 2017;153:1241–58.e29.

22. Rogolevich VV, Glushkova TV, Ponasenko AV, et al. Infective endocarditis causing native and prosthetic heart valve dysfunction. Kardiologiia 2019;59:68–77 [In Russian].

23. Jillella DV, Wisco DR. Infectious causes of stroke. Curr Opin Infect Dis 2019;32:285–92.

24. Sotero FD, Rosario M, Fonseca AC, et al. Neurological complications of infective endocarditis. Curr Neurol Neurosci Rep 2019;19:23.

25. Li JS, Sexton DJ, Mick N, et al. Proposed modifications to the Duke criteria for the diagnosis of infective endocarditis. Clin Infect Dis 2000;30:633–8.

26. Fowler VG Jr, Miro JM, Hoen B, et al. *Staphylococcus aureus* endocarditis: a consequence of medical progress. JAMA 2005;293:3012–21.

27. Lauridsen TK, Park L, Tong SY, et al. Echocardiographic findings predict in-hospital and 1-year mortality in left-sided native valve Staphylococcus aureus endocarditis: analysis from the International Collaboration on Endocarditis-Prospective Echo Cohort Study. Circ Cardiovasc Imaging 2015;8: e003397.

28. Baddour LM, Wilson WR, Bayer AS, et al. Infective endocarditis in adults: diagnosis, antimicrobial therapy, and management of complications: a scientific statement for healthcare professionals from the American Heart Association. Circulation 2015;132: 1435–86.

29. Casella F, Rana B, Casazza G, et al. The potential impact of contemporary transthoracic echocardiography on the management of patients with native valve endocarditis: a comparison with transesophageal echocardiography. Echocardiography 2009;26: 900–6.

30. Nadji G, Rusinaru D, Remadi JP, et al. Heart failure in left-sided native valve infective endocarditis: characteristics, prognosis, and results of surgical treatment. Eur J Heart Fail 2009;11:668–75.

31. Banchs J, Yusuf SW. Echocardiographic evaluation of cardiac infections. Expert Rev Cardiovasc Ther 2012;10:1–4.

32. Morguet AJ, Werner GS, Andreas S, et al. Diagnostic value of transesophageal compared with transthoracic echocardiography in suspected prosthetic valve endocarditis. Herz 1995;20: 390–8.

33. Sochowski RA, Chan KL. Implication of negative results on a monoplane transesophageal echocardiographic study in patients with suspected infective endocarditis. J Am Coll Cardiol 1993;21:216–21.

34. Daniel WG, Mugge A, Martin RP, et al. Improvement in the diagnosis of abscesses associated with endocarditis by transesophageal echocardiography. N Engl J Med 1991;324:795–800.

35. Habib G, Lancellotti P, Antunes MJ, et al. 2015 ESC guidelines for the management of infective endocarditis: the task force for the management of infective endocarditis of the European Society of Cardiology (ESC). Endorsed by: European Association for Cardio-Thoracic Surgery (EACTS), the European Association of Nuclear Medicine (EANM). Eur Heart J 2015;36:3075–128.

36. Vieira ML, Grinberg M, Pomerantzeff PM, et al. Repeated echocardiographic examinations of patients with suspected infective endocarditis. Heart 2004;90:1020–4.

37. Sanfilippo AJ, Picard MH, Newell JB, et al. Echocardiographic assessment of patients with infectious endocarditis: prediction of risk for complications. J Am Coll Cardiol 1991;18:1191–9.

38. Berdejo J, Shibayama K, Harada K, et al. Evaluation of vegetation size and its relationship with embolism in infective endocarditis: a real-time 3-dimensional transesophageal echocardiography study. Circ Cardiovasc Imaging 2014;7:149–54.

39. Liu YW, Tsai WC, Lin CC, et al. Usefulness of real-time three-dimensional echocardiography for diagnosis of infective endocarditis. Scand Cardiovasc J 2009;43:318–23.

40. Millaire A, Van Belle E, de Groote P, et al. Obstruction of the left main coronary ostium due to an aortic vegetation: survival after early surgery. Clin Infect Dis 1996;22:192–3.

41. Middlemost S, Wisenbaugh T, Meyerowitz C, et al. A case for early surgery in native left-sided endocarditis complicated by heart failure: results in 203 patients. J Am Coll Cardiol 1991;18:663–7.

42. Saikrishnan N, Kumar G, Sawaya FJ, et al. Accurate assessment of aortic stenosis: a review of diagnostic modalities and hemodynamics. Circulation 2014; 129:244–53.

43. Baumgartner H, Falk V, Bax JJ, et al. 2017 ESC/ EACTS guidelines for the management of valvular heart disease. Eur Heart J 2017;38:2739–91.

44. Kitai T, Okada Y, Shomura Y, et al. Early surgery for asymptomatic mitral regurgitation: importance of atrial fibrillation. J Heart Valve Dis 2012;21:61–70.

45. Kitai T, Okada Y, Shomura Y, et al. Timing of valve repair for severe degenerative mitral regurgitation and long-term left ventricular function. J Thorac Cardiovasc Surg 2014;148:1978–82.

46. Kitai T, Furukawa Y, Murotani K, et al. Therapeutic strategy for functional tricuspid regurgitation in patients undergoing mitral valve repair for severe mitral regurgitation. Int J Cardiol 2017;227:803–7.

47. Lopez J, Sevilla T, Vilacosta I, et al. Prognostic role of persistent positive blood cultures after initiation of antibiotic therapy in left-sided infective endocarditis. Eur Heart J 2013;34:1749–54.

48. Yoshinaga M, Niwa K, Niwa A, et al. Risk factors for in-hospital mortality during infective endocarditis in patients with congenital heart disease. Am J Cardiol 2008;101:114–8.

49. Nguyen MH, Nguyen ML, Yu VL, et al. Candida prosthetic valve endocarditis: prospective study of six cases, review of the literature. Clin Infect Dis 1996;22:262–7.

50. Fernando RJ, Johnson SD, Augoustides JG, et al. Simultaneous right-sided, left-sided infective endocarditis: management challenges in a multidisciplinary setting. J Cardiothorac Vasc Anesth 2018;32:1041–9.

51. Hitzeroth J, Beckett N, Ntuli P. An approach to a patient with infective endocarditis. S Afr Med J 2016; 106:145–50.

52. Prendergast BD, Tornos P. Surgery for infective endocarditis: who and when? Circulation 2010;121: 1141–52.

53. Anguera I, Miro JM, Vilacosta I, et al. Aorto-cavitary fistulous tract formation in infective endocarditis: clinical, echocardiographic features of 76 cases and risk factors for mortality. Eur Heart J 2005;26: 288–97.

54. Omari B, Shapiro S, Ginzton L, et al. Predictive risk factors for periannular extension of native valve endocarditis. Clinical and echocardiographic analyses. Chest 1989;96:1273–9.

55. Cosmi JE, Tunick PA, Kronzon I. Mortality in patients with paravalvular abscess diagnosed by transesophageal echocardiography. J Am Soc Echocardiogr 2004;17:766–8.

56. Molavi A. Endocarditis: recognition, management, and prophylaxis. Cardiovasc Clin 1993;23:139–74.

57. Arnett EN, Roberts WC. Valve ring abscess in active infective endocarditis. Frequency, location, and clues to clinical diagnosis from the study of 95 necropsy patients. Circulation 1976;54:140–5.

58. Bruun NE, Habib G, Thuny F, et al. Cardiac imaging in infectious endocarditis. Eur Heart J 2014;35: 624–32.

59. Pizzi MN, Roque A, Fernandez-Hidalgo N, et al. Improving the diagnosis of infective endocarditis in prosthetic valves and intracardiac devices with 18F-fluordeoxyglucose positron emission tomography/computed tomography angiography: initial results at an infective endocarditis referral center. Circulation 2015;132:1113–26.

60. Cheitlin MD, Armstrong WF, Aurigemma GP, et al. ACC/AHA/ASE 2003 guideline update for the clinical application of echocardiography: summary article: a report of the American College of Cardiology/American Heart Association Task Force on Practice Guidelines (ACC/AHA/ASE Committee to Update the 1997 guidelines for the clinical application of echocardiography). Circulation 2003;108: 1146–62.

61. Stewart WJ, Shan K. The diagnosis of prosthetic valve endocarditis by echocardiography. Semin Thorac Cardiovasc Surg 1995;7:7–12.

62. Roe MT, Abramson MA, Li J, et al. Clinical information determines the impact of transesophageal echocardiography on the diagnosis of infective endocarditis by the Duke criteria. Am Heart J 2000; 139:945–51.

63. Heiro M, Nikoskelainen J, Engblom E, et al. Neurologic manifestations of infective endocarditis: a 17-year experience in a teaching hospital in Finland. Arch Intern Med 2000;160:2781–7.

64. Steckelberg JM, Murphy JG, Ballard D, et al. Emboli in infective endocarditis: the prognostic value of echocardiography. Ann Intern Med 1991;114: 635–40.

65. De Castro S, Magni G, Beni S, et al. Role of transthoracic and transesophageal echocardiography in predicting embolic events in patients with active infective endocarditis involving native cardiac valves. Am J Cardiol 1997;80:1030–4.

66. Snygg-Martin U, Gustafsson L, Rosengren L, et al. Cerebrovascular complications in patients with left-sided infective endocarditis are common: a prospective study using magnetic resonance imaging and neurochemical brain damage markers. Clin Infect Dis 2008;47:23–30.

67. Vilacosta I, Graupner C, San Roman JA, et al. Risk of embolization after institution of antibiotic therapy for infective endocarditis. J Am Coll Cardiol 2002;39: 1489–95.

68. Thuny F, Di Salvo G, Belliard O, et al. Risk of embolism and death in infective endocarditis: prognostic value of echocardiography: a prospective multicenter study. Circulation 2005;112:69–75.

69. Nishimura RA, Otto CM, Bonow RO, et al. 2017 AHA/ACC focused update of the 2014 AHA/ACC guideline for the management of patients with valvular heart disease: a report of the American College of Cardiology/American Heart Association Task Force on Clinical Practice Guidelines. Circulation 2017; 135:e1159–95.

70. Dickerman SA, Abrutyn E, Barsic B, et al. The relationship between the initiation of antimicrobial therapy and the incidence of stroke in infective endocarditis: an analysis from the ICE Prospective Cohort Study (ICE-PCS). Am Heart J 2007;154: 1086–94.

71. Kang DH, Kim YJ, Kim SH, et al. Early surgery versus conventional treatment for infective endocarditis. N Engl J Med 2012;366:2466–73.

72. Rohmann S, Erbel R, Gorge G, et al. Clinical relevance of vegetation localization by transoesophageal echocardiography in infective endocarditis. Eur Heart J 1992;13:446–52.

73. Bayer AS, Bolger AF, Taubert KA, et al. Diagnosis and management of infective endocarditis and its complications. Circulation 1998;98:2936–48.

74. Roder BL, Wandall DA, Espersen F, et al. Neurologic manifestations in *Staphylococcus aureus* endocarditis: a review of 260 bacteremic cases in nondrug addicts. Am J Med 1997;102:379–86.

75. Ruttmann E, Willeit J, Ulmer H, et al. Neurological outcome of septic cardioembolic stroke after infective endocarditis. Stroke 2006;37:2094–9.

76. Anderson DJ, Goldstein LB, Wilkinson WE, et al. Stroke location, characterization, severity, and outcome in mitral vs aortic valve endocarditis. Neurology 2003;61:1341–6.

77. Murai R, Funakoshi S, Kaji S, et al. Outcomes of early surgery for infective endocarditis with moderate cerebral complications. J Thorac Cardiovasc Surg 2017;153:831–40.e8.

78. Goulenok T, Klein I, Mazighi M, et al. Infective endocarditis with symptomatic cerebral complications: contribution of cerebral magnetic resonance imaging. Cerebrovasc Dis 2013;35:327–36.

79. Hess A, Klein I, Iung B, et al. Brain MRI findings in neurologically asymptomatic patients with infective endocarditis. AJNR Am J Neuroradiol 2013;34:1579–84.

80. Jones HR Jr, Siekert RG. Neurological manifestations of infective endocarditis. Review of clinical and therapeutic challenges. Brain 1989;112(Pt 5):1295–315.

81. Parrino PE, Kron IL, Ross SD, et al. Does a focal neurologic deficit contraindicate operation in a patient with endocarditis? Ann Thorac Surg 1999;67:59–64.

82. Garcia-Cabrera E, Fernandez-Hidalgo N, Almirante B, et al. Neurological complications of infective endocarditis: risk factors, outcome, and impact of cardiac surgery: a multicenter observational study. Circulation 2013;127:2272–84.

83. Cooper HA, Thompson EC, Laureno R, et al. Subclinical brain embolization in left-sided infective endocarditis: results from the evaluation by MRI of the brains of patients with left-sided intracardiac solid masses (EMBOLISM) pilot study. Circulation 2009;120:585–91.

84. Klein I, Iung B, Labreuche J, et al. Cerebral microbleeds are frequent in infective endocarditis: a case-control study. Stroke 2009;40:3461–5.

85. Duval X, Iung B, Klein I, et al. Effect of early cerebral magnetic resonance imaging on clinical decisions in infective endocarditis: a prospective study. Ann Intern Med 2010;152:497–504. W175.

86. Okazaki S, Sakaguchi M, Hyun B, et al. Cerebral microbleeds predict impending intracranial hemorrhage in infective endocarditis. Cerebrovasc Dis 2011;32:483–8.

87. Murai R, Kaji S, Kitai T, et al. The clinical significance of cerebral microbleeds in infective endocarditis patients. Semin Thorac Cardiovasc Surg 2019;31:51–8.

88. Bisdas T, Teebken OE. Mycotic or infected aneurysm? Time to change the term. Eur J Vasc Endovasc Surg 2011;41:570 [author reply: 570–1].

89. Chapot R, Houdart E, Saint-Maurice JP, et al. Endovascular treatment of cerebral mycotic aneurysms. Radiology 2002;222:389–96.

90. Fukuda W, Daitoku K, Minakawa M, et al. Management of infective endocarditis with cerebral complications. Ann Thorac Cardiovasc Surg 2014;20:229–36.

91. Gordon SM, Serkey JM, Longworth DL, et al. Early onset prosthetic valve endocarditis: the Cleveland Clinic experience 1992-1997. Ann Thorac Surg 2000;69:1388–92.

92. Wolff M, Witchitz S, Chastang C, et al. Prosthetic valve endocarditis in the ICU. Prognostic factors of overall survival in a series of 122 cases and consequences for treatment decision. Chest 1995;108:688–94.

93. Tornos P, Almirante B, Olona M, et al. Clinical outcome and long-term prognosis of late prosthetic valve endocarditis: a 20-year experience. Clin Infect Dis 1997;24:381–6.

94. Lopez J, Sevilla T, Vilacosta I, et al. Clinical significance of congestive heart failure in prosthetic valve endocarditis. A multicenter study with 257 patients. Rev Esp Cardiol (Engl Ed) 2013;66:384–90.

95. Habib G, Tribouilloy C, Thuny F, et al. Prosthetic valve endocarditis: who needs surgery? A multicentre study of 104 cases. Heart 2005;91:954–9.

96. Lalani T, Chu VH, Park LP, et al. In-hospital and 1-year mortality in patients undergoing early surgery for prosthetic valve endocarditis. JAMA Intern Med 2013;173:1495–504.

97. Sandoe JA, Barlow G, Chambers JB, et al. Guidelines for the diagnosis, prevention and management of implantable cardiac electronic device infection. Report of a joint working party project on behalf of the British Society for Antimicrobial Chemotherapy (BSAC, host organization), British Heart Rhythm Society (BHRS), British Cardiovascular Society (BCS), British Heart Valve Society (BHVS), British Society for Echocardiography (BSE). J Antimicrob Chemother 2015;70:325–59.

98. Fu HX, Huang XM, Zhong LI, et al. Outcomes and complications of lead removal: can we establish a risk stratification schema for a collaborative and effective approach? Pacing Clin Electrophysiol 2015;38:1439–47.

Minimally Invasive Mitral Surgery
Patient Selection and Technique

Daniel J.P. Burns, MD, MPhil*, Per Wierup, MD, PhD, Marc Gillinov, MD

KEYWORDS

• Minimally invasive • Mitral valve • Thoracotomy • Robotic-assisted

KEY POINTS

• Patient selection is critical to successful minimally invasive mitral valve procedures.
• A formal assessment based on select echocardiographic and computed tomography features guides the selection process.
• Patient safety is the number one guiding principle.
• Appropriately selected patients should be able to undergo the full range of mitral valve repair or replacement techniques.

INTRODUCTION

Although minimally invasive approaches have become standard of care in many surgical specialties, cardiac surgery has traditionally lagged behind in the adoption of minimally invasive techniques, apart from certain highly specialized centers. Owing to excellent exposure and a high degree of procedural control, the sternotomy is the default for most cardiac surgical procedures. With respect to minimally invasive surgery, the guiding principle is that it is preferable, provided the same or better results can be achieved. However, as we move to a less invasive approach, we necessarily relinquish a certain degree of control. The balance between access and control is fundamental to ensuring patient safety and excellent results.

Mitral valve repair surgery is particularly amenable to a minimally invasive approach, with the expected benefits identical to a conventional approach: superior survival and decreased risks of thromboembolism, endocarditis, anticoagulant-related hemorrhage, and reintervention relative to valve replacement.[1–5] Several approaches have been developed in the last 25 years, most of which

continue to be used in some capacity today. The spectrum of minimally invasive mitral valve approaches includes partial sternotomy, right mini-thoracotomy, and robotic assisted. Of these techniques, robotic-assisted mitral valve repair is the approach favored by the Cleveland Clinic for patients with isolated degenerative mitral valve disease. In this article, we briefly describe the different minimally invasive mitral valve surgical approaches. Building on this analysis, we discuss the process of patient selection, procedure performance, technical challenges, and clinical outcomes in robotic assisted minimally invasive mitral valve surgery.

History and Development

Highly specialized institutions began describing minimally invasive approaches to the mitral valve in the mid-1990s. These procedures began with partial sternotomy or parasternal access.[6–8] The parasternal approach has since been abandoned, but the partial sternotomy approach is still in use. Dr Carpentier first described a thoracotomy-based approach with video assistance in 1996.[9] This approach evolved to include an endoaortic balloon occlusion device and port access

Department of Thoracic and Cardiovascular Surgery, Cleveland Clinic, 9500 Euclid Avenue / J4-1, Cleveland, OH 44195, USA
* Corresponding author.
E-mail address: burnsd@ccf.org

Cardiol Clin 39 (2021) 211–220
https://doi.org/10.1016/j.ccl.2021.01.003
0733-8651/21/© 2021 Elsevier Inc. All rights reserved.

cardiology.theclinics.com

technology.[10] The minithoracotomy approach has more recently evolved to include a totally endoscopic approach with stereoscopic visualization, rivalling surgical robotics for degrees of visualization and invasiveness.[11,12]

Adapting surgical robotics to cardiac surgery has been, in our opinion, the largest leap forward in minimally invasive mitral valve surgery. The minithoracotomy approach relies on long shafted instruments and video assistance, necessarily limited by the lack of depth perception with 2-dimensional video and limited dexterity with long shafted surgical instruments. Robotic assistance avoids these limitations. There have now been several generations of surgical robotic systems. These devices humbly began with a voice-activated camera arm, and have progressed through multiple generations of telemanipulation systems. The current generation system is the DaVinci Xi (Intuitive Surgical Inc., Sunnyvale, CA), the fourth generation of DaVinci systems. This system provides superior visualization of the mitral valve, with a highly magnified, high-definition 3-dimensional view. With the robotic approach, dexterity is unrivaled. Telemanipulation with tremor reduction provides the surgical robot with the capability of 7° of freedom. The surgeon is provided with a full, stable, unimpinged range of motion. The nonrobotic, totally endoscopic approach with stereoscopic visualization may rival the robotic approach, but the dexterity advantage in current surgical robotics is undeniable.

Intimately involved in the evolution of cardiac surgery, the first robotic-assisted cardiac procedure was described by Dr Carpentier in 1998; this procedure was the repair of an atrial septal defect.[13] Adapting surgical robotics to mitral valve repair, using the early DaVinci system, was pioneered by Dr Chitwood in 2000. Dr Chitwood and his team were able to use the full range of mitral valve repair techniques and demonstrated excellent results.[14] The experience of Dr Chitwood has been the model from which modern robotic mitral valve surgery has evolved.

CENTRAL DISCUSSION: ROBOTIC-ASSISTED MITRAL VALVE SURGERY
Patient Selection

Most patients with isolated degenerative disease can have their mitral valve repaired using a robotic approach, although, in practice, not all patients should. Patient selection is essential to the success of robotic assisted mitral valve surgery. Complications most commonly stem from improper patient selection. The Cleveland Clinic has adopted a relatively conservative screening algorithm

for robotic-assisted mitral valve surgery, which has helped to decrease incident complications (**Fig. 1**).[15] We consider patients with significant coronary artery disease requiring revascularization, or a prior sternotomy, precluded from a robotic approach. Regarding coronary disease, although minimally invasive coronary artery bypass grafting, or even hybrid revascularization could be attempted in the setting of a robotic-assisted mitral valve operation, this technique greatly increases both operative time and complexity, and would likely be executed more safely and efficiently from a sternotomy approach. Regarding the patient with a prior sternotomy, we perform reoperations almost universally through a sternotomy approach to maximize patient safety and surgical control. The patient with a high body mass index should still be considered for robotic-assisted mitral valve surgery. However, meticulous care should be taken with incision, port placement, and ensuring postprocedure hemostasis, because bleeding complications can be challenging to address.

In the absence of these factors, the decision of whether to offer a robotic approach depends on the results of preoperative imaging studies, with every patient considered undergoing a preoperative transthoracic echocardiogram and contrast-enhanced computed tomography (CT) scan (see **Fig. 1**).[15]

Echocardiographic Features

Echocardiographic features influencing the decision to offer robotic assisted mitral surgery are mitral annular calcification (MAC), aortic insufficiency, significant left or right ventricular dysfunction, and severe pulmonary hypertension. MAC complicates the performance of an adequate complete repair; if required, MAC debridement can greatly increase the complexity and surgical risk of a mitral valve repair. This process not only prolongs the operation, but can predispose to injury. The requirement to debride and patch the mitral annulus, and the associated risk of annular complications, steers us away from a minimally invasive approach when confronted with significant MAC. Even if debridement and patching are not required, the annulus is stiffened and can cause problems with exposure. Patients with severe MAC are best served by a sternotomy-based approach, although those with mild MAC may be candidates for robotic surgery and the MAC burden should be confirmed by the preoperative CT scan. For these reasons, it is essential to understand the condition of the mitral annulus before the operation.

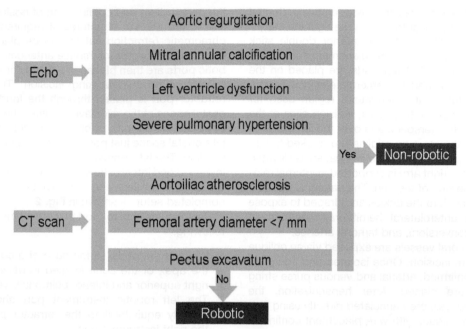

Fig. 1. Algorithm for patient selection in robotic-assisted mitral valve surgery.

We favor antegrade single dose Del Nido cardioplegia for robotic-assisted mitral surgery. Greater than mild aortic insufficiency makes antegrade cardioplegia problematic, and increases the risk of both ventricular distension and inadequate myocardial protection. That being said, some groups rely on percutaneous retrograde cardioplegia cannulas during robotic surgery; great care must be taken to ensure that these cannulas do not become dislodged during surgery, particularly in the patient with aortic insufficiency that is moderate or greater.

We believe that a sternotomy approach should be used for patients with severe left or right ventricular dysfunction to optimize both myocardial protection and operative time. If there are inadequate or inconclusive results from the transthoracic echocardiogram, a preoperative transesophageal echocardiogram (TEE) is completed for clarification.

Computed Tomography Features

A contrast-enhanced CT scan of the chest, abdomen, and pelvis informs cannulation and perfusion strategies, as well as an understanding of the patient's thoracic anatomy for incision and port placement. Significant aortoiliac atherosclerosis, particularly if there is soft plaque present, precludes safe retrograde perfusion via the femoral artery, increasing the risk of cerebrovascular events.[16] Small femoral arteries (<7 mm diameter) or heavily calcified femoral arteries can

preclude the safe insertion of an adequately sized femoral arterial cannula, or the safe side grafting of the femoral artery. The CT scan will define which side is preferable for femoral access, based on areas of disease and/or tortuosity. Aberrant vascular anatomy influencing perfusion strategy (discontinuous inferior vena cava, persistent left superior vena cava, or a retroesophageal left subclavian artery) will be identified with a preoperative CT scan, and often precludes a robotic-assisted approach.

Patients with significant pectus excavatum should also be addressed with a sternotomy-based approach. The issue here becomes exposure of the valve itself. With the anterior–posterior diameter of the chest focally decreased , the ability to retract the interatrial septum to expose the mitral valve is compromised. With inadequate exposure, the safety and adequacy of the operation may be compromised. Because the goal of robotic-assisted mitral repair is a repair of the same quality and durability as one performed by sternotomy, exposure concerns are especially problematic.

Anesthesia and Perfusion

To achieve single lung ventilation, intubation is completed using a double lumen endotracheal tube or a single lumen tube with bronchial blocker. A TEE probe is placed in every case to confirm preoperative findings, better define the mitral anatomy, guide the peripheral cannulation, and confirm adequate results postoperatively. Central venous access is obtained via the right internal jugular vein, followed by an inferior double stick catheter to facilitate wire placement for bicaval cannulation. Defibrillator pads are placed on the right posterior and left anterolateral hemithorax, avoiding the right anterolateral region used for port placement. Interspaces, incision sites at the lateral fourth interspace and over the femoral vessels, and the sternum midline are marked before positioning. The right side of the patient is elevated 30°, and the right arm is supported in internal rotation off the side of the bed. The patient is prepped from the neck to the ankles and draped to expose the right anterolateral hemithorax, sternum (in case of conversion), and femoral arteries.

The femoral vessels are exposed via an oblique 2- to 3-cm incision. Once isolated and adequate size is confirmed, arterial and venous purse string sutures are placed. After heparinization, the femoral vessels are cannulated directly using Seldinger technique, with wire placement confirmed by TEE. The femoral venous cannula is placed so that the tip sits 2 to 3 cm into the superior vena cava. After TEE confirmation of the arterial wire in the aorta, the arterial cannula is placed such that the tip sits in the distal abdominal aorta or iliac artery. Inadequately sized femoral arteries can lead to inadequate systemic flows, as well as to distal limb ischemia. To mitigate this feature, alternative perfusion strategies must be considered. Perfusion via a femoral artery side graft will prevent distal limb ischemia, although the artery still must be adequately sized to support systemic flow. Although not used at our institution, antegrade perfusion via direct aortic cannulation or axillary artery cannulation has been described. Our approach, however, has been to abandon the robotic-assisted approach when faced with inadequately sized femoral arteries.

In patients with a body surface area of 2.0 m^2 or more, a bicaval venous cannulation approach is used. The inferior right internal jugular catheter is used to pass a guide wire into the right atrium under TEE guidance. An additional 15F to 18F venous cannula is then placed percutaneously into the superior vena cava.

Port Placement

After confirmation of femoral vessel size, the right lung is deflated and a 3- to 4-cm working incision is created in the right fourth intercostal space, bisecting the anterior axillary line. In women, the right breast is retracted medially and superiorly, so the incision can be placed in the breast crease. Gentle spreading of the ribs allows visualization of

the pericardium and confirmation of position relative to the cardiac structures. If required, a diaphragmatic retraction suture can be placed and run out in an inferior interspace anteriorly. The robotic ports are then placed in a triangular configuration around the working incision. The atrial retractor port is placed through the fourth intercostal space at the midclavicular line. The right robotic instrument arm is placed through the sixth intercostal space just posterior to the anterior axillary line. The left robotic instrument arm is placed in the second intercostal space roughly in between the anterior axillary and midclavicular lines. The completed setup is shown in **Fig. 2**.

Useful guidelines for port placement include the following:

1. Imagine the ports as the base of a cone, with the apex of the cone located in between the right superior and inferior pulmonary veins.
2. The left robotic instrument port should be roughly equilateral to the retractor port and the right instrument port.
3. The distance between port sites may need to be increased or decreased based on the patient's body habitus to optimize robotic arm range of motion and avoid arm conflicts.

Clamping and Cardioplegia

Once port placement has been completed, cardiopulmonary bypass is commenced and the heart is decompressed; the patient is cooled to 30°C. Through the working incision, the pericardial fat is excised, and the pericardium is opened longitudinally starting near the diaphragm and extending cranially to expose the aorta. This incision should

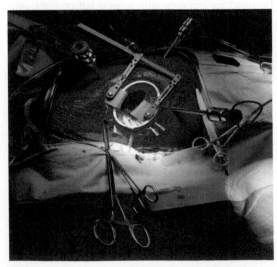

Fig. 2. Final patient setup before robot docking.

be initiated at least 3 cm anterior to the phrenic nerve. It is useful to mark the phrenic nerve in ink to ensure it is avoided. Autologous pericardium is harvested from the anterior aspect of this incision. Pericardial retraction sutures are placed on the posterior aspect of the pericardial incision in the region of the superior vena cava and inferior vena cava, and the sutures are taken out posteriorly through the chest wall.

Two strategies have been described to achieve aortic occlusion and subsequent cardioplegia delivery in minimally invasive mitral valve operations. The first involves placing a separate aortic root cannula for cardioplegia delivery and aortic root venting, along with a transthoracic clamp. The cardioplegia cannula is placed via the working incision. The transthoracic clamp is placed through the third interspace in the midaxillary line. The clamp lies in the transverse sinus and is oriented so the concavity of the clamp is directed cranially. Care must be taken to avoid the pulmonary trunk, left atrial appendage, and left main coronary artery when clamping the aorta. Proper positioning of the transthoracic clamp is essential. This technique will avoid excess tension on the aorta and minimize the rotation and on the aorta after clamping. Additionally, the clamp must lie posterior enough such that the left robotic arm does not exert undue pressure on the clamp during the procedure, predisposing to aortic injury.

The second strategy uses endoaortic balloon occlusion with integrated cardioplegia delivery and venting capability, all facilitated by a catheter introduced via the femoral artery. Balloon positioning is confirmed by TEE and, in some institutions, by fluoroscopy. Bilateral upper extremity arterial lines are required, because the balloon may migrate distally, which can be detected by a decrease in the right upper extremity blood pressure. Because of the possibility of the balloon becoming malpositioned, placing a retrograde cardioplegia catheter via the internal jugular vein is prudent to ensure adequate myocardial protection. Using the endoaortic balloon allows the working port to be reduced in size or eliminated in a totally endoscopic approach. However, it increases procedural complexity and costs.[17] In addition to being somewhat unpredictable and temperamental, the endoaortic balloon also seems to increase the risk of aortic dissection.[18]

Our preferred approach is to use a transthoracic clamp and deliver direct antegrade cardioplegia via the aortic root. We use single dose Del Nido cardioplegia at 20 mL/kg. Additional cardioplegia is given at 60 minutes if the cross-clamp time is expected to exceed 90 minutes. This strategy, one may argue, is not fundamentally different in terms of setup than a nonrobotic minithoracotomy approach. However, this assertion is not incorrect. The advantages are retained in visualization and dexterity, and we believe the transthoracic clamp approach to be safe and predictable. Also, it allows for valve replacement without sternotomy conversion if repair is unsuccessful, although the working incision may need to be extended to accommodate a prosthetic.

Mitral Valve Repair

All advanced mitral valve repair techniques used in sternotomy approaches can be used with a robotic-assisted approach.[19] Only minor modifications are required to accommodate the robotic instruments, and we have described several techniques that have been developed to improve surgical efficiency.[20] The mitral valve is approached through a left atriotomy, using the robotic atrial retractor to optimize valve exposure. As with any mitral valve repair, initial valve inspection takes place, and the repair technique is tailored to the specific valve lesion(s) and morphology.

Posterior leaflet resection and the creation of artificial chordae are both routinely performed with robotic assistance. Narrow regions of prolapse can be addressed with a triangular resection using robotic-adapted scissors and Resano forceps. Interrupted figure-of-eight 4-0 polypropylene sutures re-approximate free leaflet edges. Excessively tall and bulky regions of prolapse are managed by quadrangular resection and sliding plasty, again using 4-0 polypropylene suture for valve reconstruction. This eliminates the prolapse and decreases the height of the posterior leaflet, reducing the risk of systolic anterior motion. The remaining cases of posterior prolapse are managed with artificial chordae.

Posterior neochordae are fashioned using CV-4 polytetrafluoroethylene (PTFE) sutures. These are premeasured based on the affected leaflet, knotted at the tail end, and marked at 1.5 cm from the terminal knot (**Fig. 3**). This marking facilitates an estimation of the chordal length. The PTFE suture is first passed through the valve leaflet (atrial to ventricular). It is then passed through the fibrous region of the corresponding papillary muscle, then back through the valve leaflet (ventricular to atrial), approximately 1 cm from the knotted tail. The suture is then passed twice more (ventricular to atrial) to finish adjacent to the knotted tail on the atrial side. The chord length is then adjusted to eliminate prolapse and ensure a favorable zone of coaptation, and the suture is tied. Care is taken to ensure that the chordae are adequately short to mitigate the risk of

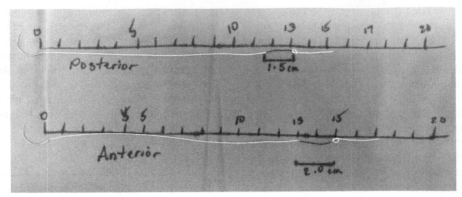

Fig. 3. PTFE neochordae constructed based on the affected valve leaflet.

systolic anterior motion. For a typical P2 prolapse, 2 sets of chordae are used. As required, deep indentations between adjacent P1/2 or P2/3 scallops are closed with interrupted figure-of-eight 4-0 polypropylene sutures. Alternatively, these indentations can be spanned by neochordae. We prefer to use free-hand chordal adjustment, although the use of premeasured neochordae is equally effective.[21]

For the repair of an isolated anterior leaflet prolapse, artificial chordae are preferred. The technique is identical to that previously described, although the PTFE sutures are longer and marked at 2 cm from the terminal knot (see **Fig. 3**). Two sets of chords are fashioned. These chords are oriented on either side of the leaflet midline and are anchored posteriorly to the corresponding lateral or medial papillary muscle. Chord length is adjusted such that prolapse is eliminated and the coaptation zone is moved posteriorly. An isolated A1 or A3 prolapse is typically corrected with commissuroplasty.

Bileaflet prolapse can be managed with a combination of techniques. A true Barlow valve with an exceptional amount of redundant tissue can be managed with a posterior resection and 2 sets of anterior chords. Recently, we have adopted a 4 chords approach to these complex valves.[22] The anterior leaflet is addressed first to optimize papillary muscle exposure, followed by the posterior leaflet. In all cases, each chord corresponds to the medial or lateral aspect of each leaflet, and does not cross the midline. Neochordae are anchored to posterior aspects of the corresponding papillary muscles. Indentations in the posterior leaflet are managed as described previously. Great care is taken to optimize leaflet height. Neochordae must both eliminate prolapse and also move the coaptation zone adequately posterior to mitigate against systolic anterior motion. To this end, posterior leaflet neochordae are left intentionally short (<1 cm).

In line with standard mitral valve repair practices, all repairs should include an annuloplasty. Regardless of the annuloplasty device used, excellent results can be expected.[23,24] We prefer a flexible band annuloplasty owing to its ease of manipulation within the left atrium. There are 3 methods of annuloplasty fixation available: interrupted sutures manually tied with a knot pushing device, interrupted sutures fixed with titanium fasteners, and a running suture fixation. The running annuloplasty uses three 2-0 braided polyester sutures measuring 16, 14, and 9 cm. Each has a preknotted tail to anchor the suture, decreasing the number of robotically tied knots required (**Fig. 4**). Beginning at the posteromedial trigone, the suture is run clockwise to the midportion of the annulus, tied to the second suture, and the second suture continued until the suture reaches the anterolateral trigone. At this point, a third suture is passed though the annuloplasty band, anchored to the anterolateral trigone, and brought back through the band. This third suture is then tied in close proximity to the second. All knot tying is completed with the robotic instruments. This technique was developed at the Cleveland Clinic to optimize surgical efficiency for robotic cases.[20] On completion of the annuloplasty, the valve repair is then tested using conventional saline insufflation.

Left atrial closure is simplified by using 2 CV-4 PTFE sutures fashioned with small loops at each tail and 5-8 pretied knots (**Fig. 5**).[20] This loop creates a snare at the terminal end of the suture, avoiding additional robotic knot tying. One suture is used at each terminal end of the left atriotomy, and run toward the center. A drop suction is placed across the mitral valve before left atrial closure, and removed once the heart begins to eject during weaning from cardiopulmonary bypass, expediting de-airing.

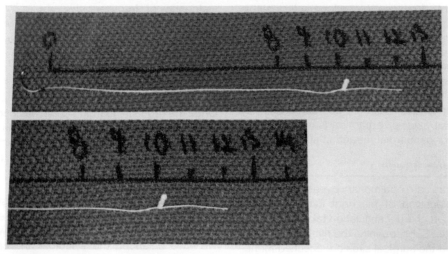

Fig. 4. Preknotted sutures for running mitral annuloplasty.

PITFALLS AND CHALLENGES
Learning Curve

Any mitral valve surgeon can transfer to the robotic platform, although the robotic platform presents several challenges. A lack of tactile feedback requires the surgeon to pay exceptionally close attention to surrounding tissues, which are susceptible to injury. This lack of feedback can also lead to broken sutures while suturing or tying. Although visualization and dexterity are superior using the robotic platform, the surgeon must necessarily relearn how to angle/pass needles and manipulate instruments, because the telemanipulation system does not exactly mirror the movements used in open surgery. Similarly, knot tying can be quite challenging when beginning to use the robotic platform given the reasons highlighted elsewhere in this article.

Equally important is team training and experience. A dedicated robotically assisted cardiac surgery team is recommended, if not essential, requiring dedicated members from anesthesia, nursing, and perfusion who are experienced and comfortable with the procedure. A bedside surgeon is required as well, who must be comfortable with both the robotic technology and the ability to pass sutures, help expose, and generally facilitate the operation. The entire team must negotiate the requisite learning curve. With experience, comfort with the platform improves, as does operative efficiency, which steadily improves until reaching a plateau at approximately 150 to 200 cases.[15,25] Simulation, as an evolving adjunct, helps to decrease this learning curve.[26]

Intraoperative Injury

Cardiac structures are uniquely susceptible to injury during a robotic-assisted procedure owing to placement of the requisite instruments and their interactions during the case. Transthoracic clamping carries the risk of aortic, pulmonary artery, left atrial appendage, or left main coronary artery injury. The transverse sinus must be adequately visualized while placing the clamp to mitigate injury to any of these structures. The transthoracic clamp can also be inadvertently manipulated and torqued by the left robotic instrument if the port is placed with inadequate clearance of the cross-clamp, increasing the risk of aortic injury. Similarly, the left instrument can interact with the antegrade cardioplegia cannula and cause aortic injury.

An endoaortic occlusion balloon can mitigate the risk of pulmonary artery, left atrial appendage, and left main coronary artery injury, as well as eliminate the risk of inadvertent aortic manipulation. However, the endoaortic occlusion balloon seems to increase the risk of aortic dissection and conversion to sternotomy.[17,18] Additionally, aortic occlusion and cardioplegia can be

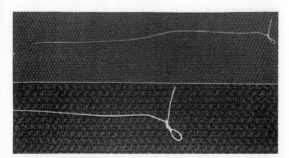

Fig. 5. PTFE suture with end snare, used for left atriotomy closure.

unpredictable, because the balloon is less stable and prone to dislodging.[27]

Phrenic nerve injury can be mitigated by incising the pericardium at least 3 cm anterior to the phrenic nerve. Marking the phrenic nerve in ink before incising the pericardium serves as a useful technique for avoiding the nerve. The risk of phrenic injury can further be decreased by ensuring that excessive traction is not placed on the posterior pericardial retraction sutures.

Postoperative Bleeding

Weaning from cardiopulmonary bypass typically requires reexpansion of the right lung. Protamine administration and decannulation take place in the usual fashion. Subsequently, the right lung is again deflated and the surgical sites are checked for hemostasis. Major surgical sites (atriotomy, cardioplegia cannula site, pericardial edge, and pericardial fat) are examined under direct vision, with hemostasis achieved using extra sutures or cautery as appropriate. An endoscope is inserted through the atrial retractor port and the left and right instrument ports are removed. Port sites are examined endoscopically and hemostasis is achieved with cautery as required. The atrial retractor port is then removed and the endoscope is inserted through the working port to examine this port site in the same manner. Chest tube drainage is achieved using the right instrument port site.

Meticulous care must be taken with hemostasis, as with any cardiac surgical case. A low threshold to return to the operating room to address postoperative bleeding should be adopted. Prevention is the best way to address postoperative bleeding, because visualization, exposure, and repair can be quite challenging in the context of postoperative hemorrhage in the robotic-assisted minimal access patient.

CLINICAL OUTCOMES

Since the early 2000s, robotic-assisted mitral valve surgery has consistently shown excellent results.[14,27] The entire spectrum of mitral repair techniques are possible.[14,15,28] Cardiopulmonary bypass and cross-clamp times are longer than for sternotomy, especially in the early stages of robotic adoption, but this does not seem to translate into an increase in morbidity or mortality.[28] Intensive care unit and total hospital length of stay are decreased and return to work time is improved.[28–30] Incident stroke and operative mortality consistently measure at less than 1% in major series.[28,31,32] With adoption of the described screening algorithm, the Cleveland Clinic was able achieve a 50% relative decrease our

incidence of intraoperative stroke.[15] Infectious complications are similarly low.[15,28,32] Finally, and very important to the patient, the cosmetic result is excellent.

SUMMARY

Once the requisite learning curve has been negotiated, robotic-assisted mitral surgery is safe and effective, producing results of the same quality compared with a sternotomy-based approach. The inevitable reality is that as one becomes less invasive, complexity is increased, and control is relinquished. Using the approaches described for patient selection as well as procedure execution, in robotic assisted mitral valve repair, we believe we have balanced these factors and can offer a safe, predictable, and durable complete repair.

CLINICS CARE POINTS

- Patient safety and repair quality are the 2 main guiding principles in minimally invasive mitral valve surgery.
- Formal echocardiographic and CT assessment is essential to proper patient selection, mitigating surgical risk and making the correct intervention possible via minimal access.
- In minimally invasive mitral valve surgery, all typical mitral valve repair techniques are possible, along with replacement.
- Although we favor the robotic-assisted approach, the general principles are the same between all right chest approaches.
- With any minimally invasive approach to mitral valve surgery, team experience is essential, although there will be a necessary learning curve to overcome.

DISCLOSURE

D.J.P. Burns is a consultant for Medtronic. P. Wierup is a consultant to Medtronic, Edwards Lifesciences, and CryoLife. A.M. Gillinov is a consultant to Medtronic, Edwards Lifesciences, Abbott, CryoLife, Johnson and Johnson, AtriCure, and ClearFlow; and has a right to equity from ClearFlow.

REFERENCES

1. David TE, David CM, Tsang W, et al. Long-term results of mitral valve repair for regurgitation due to

leaflet prolapse. J Am Coll Cardiol 2019;74(8):
1044–53.

2. David TE, Armstrong S, McCrindle BW, et al. Late
outcomes of mitral valve repair for mitral regurgitation due to degenerative disease. Circulation 2013;
127(14):1485–92.

3. Gillinov AM, Blackstone EH, Nowicki ER, et al. Valve
repair versus valve replacement for degenerative
mitral valve disease. J Thorac Cardiovasc Surg
2008;135(4):885–93, 893.e1-2.

4. Suri RM, Schaff HV, Dearani JA, et al. Survival
advantage and improved durability of mitral repair
for leaflet prolapse subsets in the current era. Ann
Thorac Surg 2006;82(3):819–26.

5. Braunberger E, Deloche A, Berrebi A, et al. Very
long-term results (more than 20 years) of valve
repair with Carpentier's techniques in nonrheumatic
mitral valve insufficiency. Circulation 2001;
104(SUPPL. 1):8–11.

6. Svensson LG, D'Agostino RS. "J" incision minimal-
access valve operations. Ann Thorac Surg 1998;
66(3):1110–2.

7. Navia JL, Cosgrove DM. Minimally invasive mitral
valve operations. Ann Thorac Surg 1996;62(5):
1542–4.

8. Doty DB, DiRusso GB, Doty JR. Full spectrum cardiac surgery through a minimal incision: mini-
sternotomy (lower half) technique. Ann Thorac
Surg 1998;65(2):573–7.

9. Carpentier A, Loulmet D, Carpentier A, et al. [Open
heart operation under videosurgery and mini-
thoracotomy. First case (mitral valvuloplasty) oper-
ated with success]. C R Acad Sci 1996;319(3):
219–23. Available at: http://www.ncbi.nlm.nih.gov/
pubmed/8761668.

10. Mohr FW, Falk V, Diegeler A, et al. Minimally invasive port-access mitral valve surgery. J Thorac Cardiovasc Surg 1998;115(3):567–74 [discussion:
574–6].

11. Van Praet KM, Stamm C, Sündermann SH, et al.
Minimally invasive surgical mitral valve repair: state
of the art review. Interv Cardiol (London, England)
2018;13(1):14–9.

12. Westhofen S, Conradi L, Deuse T, et al. A matched
pairs analysis of non-rib-spreading, fully endoscopic, mini-incision technique versus conventional
mini-thoracotomy for mitral valve repair. Eur J
Cardio-thoracic Surg 2016;50(6):1181–7.

13. Carpentier A, Loulmet D, Aupècle B, et al. [Com-
puter assisted open heart surgery. First case oper-
ated on with success]. C R Acad Sci 1998;321(5):
437–42. Available at: http://www.ncbi.nlm.nih.gov/
pubmed/9766192.

14. Chitwood WR, Rodriguez E, Chu MWA, et al. Robotic mitral valve repairs in 300 patients: a single-
center experience. J Thorac Cardiovasc Surg
2008;136(2):436–41.

15. Gillinov AM, Mihaljevic T, Javadikasgari H, et al.
Early results of robotically assisted mitral valve surgery: analysis of the first 1000 cases. J Thorac Cardiovasc Surg 2018;155(1):82–91.e2.

16. Burns DJ, Birla R, Vohra HA. Clinical outcomes
associated with retrograde arterial perfusion in minimally invasive mitral valve surgery: a systematic review. Perfusion 2020. https://doi.org/10.1177/
0267659120929181. 267659120929181.

17. Khan H, Hadjittofi C, Uzzaman M, et al. External
aortic clamping versus endoaortic balloon occlusion
in minimally invasive cardiac surgery: a systematic
review and meta-analysis. Interact Cardiovasc
Thorac Surg 2018;1–7. https://doi.org/10.1093/
icvts/ivy016.

18. Rival PM, Moore THM, McAleenan A, et al. Transthoracic clamp versus endoaortic balloon occlusion in
minimally invasive mitral valve surgery: a systematic
review and meta-analysis. Eur J Cardiothorac Surg
2019;0:1–11.

19. Chemtob RA, Wierup P, Mick S, et al. Choosing the
"Best" surgical techniques for mitral valve repair:
lessons from the literature. J Card Surg 2019;
717–27. https://doi.org/10.1111/jocs.14089.

20. Malas T, Mick S, Wierup P, et al. Five maneuvers to
facilitate faster robotic mitral valve repair. Semin
Thorac Cardiovasc Surg 2019;31(1):48–50.

21. Seeburger J, Borger MA, Falk V, et al. Gore-Tex loop
implantation for mitral valve prolapse: the Leipzig
loop technique. Oper Tech Thorac Cardiovasc
Surg 2008;13(2):83–90.

22. Chemtob RA, Mick S, Gillinov M, et al. Repair of bileaflet prolapse in Barlow syndrome: the 4-chord
technique. J Card Surg 2019;605–9. https://doi.
org/10.1111/jocs.14078.

23. Chang BC, Youn YN, Ha JW, et al. Long-term clinical
results of mitral valvuloplasty using flexible and rigid
rings: a prospective and randomized study.
J Thorac Cardiovasc Surg 2007;133(4):995–1003.

24. Chee T, Haston R, Togo A, et al. Is a flexible mitral annuloplasty ring superior to a semi-rigid or rigid ring in
terms of improvement in symptoms and survival?
Interact Cardiovasc Thorac Surg 2008;7(3):477–84.

25. Goodman A, Koprivanac M, Kelava M, et al. Robotic
mitral valve repair: the learning curve. Innovations
(Phila). 2017;12(6):390–7.

26. Valdis M, Chu MWA, Schlachta C, et al. Evaluation of
robotic cardiac surgery simulation training: a randomized controlled trial. J Thorac Cardiovasc Surg
2016;151(6):1498–505.e2.

27. Modi P, Hassan A, Chitwood WR. Minimally invasive
mitral valve surgery: a systematic review and meta-analysis. Eur J Cardio-thoracic Surg 2008;34(5):943–52.

28. Suri RM, Burkhart HM, Daly RC, et al. Robotic mitral
valve repair for all prolapse subsets using techniques identical to open valvuloplasty: establishing
the benchmark against which percutaneous

interventions should be judged. J Thorac Cardiovasc Surg 2011;142(5):970–9.

29. Paul S, Isaacs AJ, Jalbert J, et al. A population-based analysis of robotic-assisted mitral valve repair. Ann Thorac Surg 2015;99(5):1546–53.

30. Suri RM, Antiel RM, Burkhart HM, et al. Quality of life after early mitral valve repair using conventional and robotic approaches. Ann Thorac Surg 2012;93(3):761–9.

31. Nifong LW, Rodriguez E, Chitwood WR. 540 consecutive robotic mitral valve repairs including concomitant atrial fibrillation cryoablation. Ann Thorac Surg 2012;94(1):38–42 [discussion: 43].

32. Murphy DA, Moss E, Binongo J, et al. The expanding role of endoscopic robotics in mitral valve surgery: 1,257 consecutive procedures. Ann Thorac Surg 2015;100(5):1675–82.

Current and Future Application of Transcatheter Mitral Valve Replacement

Vinayak Nagaraja, MBBS, MS, MMed (Clin Epi), FRACP[a], Samir R. Kapadia, MD[a], Amar Krishnaswamy, MD[b],*

KEYWORDS

• Mitral annular calcification • Transcatheter mitral valve replacement • Mitral regurgitation

KEY POINTS

- Transcatheter mitral valve in valve is a safe and effective procedure for most patients with a degenerated bioprosthetic valve.
- Transcatheter mitral valve-in-ring/valve-in-mitral annular calcification outcomes are suboptimal and are reserved for patients at high or extreme surgical risk.
- Laceration of the anterior mitral leaflet to prevent left ventricular outflow tract obstruction and alcohol septal ablation are effective strategies to prevent left ventricular outflow tract obstruction.
- Several transcatheter mitral valve replacement (TMVR) device trials are underway and the ideal device is yet to be found for native TMVR.

INTRODUCTION

Transcatheter device therapy has revolutionized the way valvular heart disease has been managed in the last decade.[1–5] The landscape in transcatheter mitral valve interventions specifically has changed dramatically with randomized trial data showing the safety and efficacy of the MitraClip (Abbott Vascular, Minneapolis, MN) for patients with primary and secondary mitral regurgitation (MR).[3,6,7] However, this technology is not suitable for a large fraction of patients, including those with a failing bioprosthetic mitral valve, recurrent MR after prior ring annuloplasty, and significant mitral annular calcification (MAC) accompanying either MR or mitral stenosis (MS). Often this cohort of patients has comorbid conditions that make them not suitable for cardiac valve surgery. Transcatheter

mitral valve replacement (TMVR) may therefore be a reasonable option in patients considered high risk for conventional mitral valve surgery (replacement or repair).

This article highlights various aspects of TMVR, including the evidence, current and upcoming devices, and mitigation strategies for complications post-TMVR.

ANATOMIC CHALLENGES OF THE MITRAL VALVE

The mitral valve annulus is a dynamic, saddlelike structure that is supported by a complex subvalvular apparatus. Wide variations in pathophysiology are seen, including but not limited to MAC, functional/primary MR, MS, and mixed mitral valve disease. The heterogeneous structure of the mitral

Funding: Nil.

[a] Department of Cardiovascular Medicine, Cleveland Clinic Foundation, 9500 Euclid Avenue, Cleveland, OH 44195, USA; [b] Interventional Cardiology, Sones Cardiac Catheterization Laboratories, Interventional Cardiology Fellowship, Department of Cardiovascular Medicine, Cleveland Clinic Foundation, 9500 Euclid Avenue, Cleveland, OH 44195, USA

* Corresponding author.

E-mail address: krishna2@ccf.org

Cardiol Clin 39 (2021) 221–232
https://doi.org/10.1016/j.ccl.2021.01.006

valve poses many challenges, such as device anchoring, delivery, position, and paravalvular regurgitation. Another anatomic challenge is the proximity to the aortic valve, and TMVR can be complicated by severe left ventricular outflow tract (LVOT) obstruction, which can potentially be life threatening.

PREPROCEDURAL IMAGING
Echocardiography

Transthoracic echocardiography (TTE) and transesophageal echocardiography (TEE) are good initial imaging modalities to evaluate mitral valve pathophysiology. A thorough discussion of the contemporary role of echocardiography in assessing patients with MR is beyond the scope of this article and has been well covered in various state-of-the-art review articles.[8,9] Briefly, they provide valuable information regarding left and right ventricular size and function, pulmonary pressure, mitral valve annulus, annular calcification, subvalvular apparatus, and papillary muscles. Three-dimensional echocardiography is an extremely useful tool providing greater details regarding the mitral valve disorder and pathophysiology, especially when combined with the use of multiplanar reconstruction.

Some of the echocardiographic features that may favor TMVR rather than transcatheter mitral valve repair are commissural MR, broad MR jet across the coaptation line or with a large coaptation gap, mitral valve area less than 3.5 cm^2, multiple prolapsing segments, mixed mitral valve disease with predominant MS, severe calcification at the grasping zone, short (<7 mm) and significantly tethered posterior mitral valve leaflet, and a cleft or perforation. In analyzing patients for valve in valve (ViV) or valve in surgical mitral ring (ViR) TMVR, special consideration should be given to ruling out periprosthetic regurgitation.

Multidetector Cardiac Computed Tomography

Multidetector cardiac computed tomography is imperative for preoperative planning of TMVR. Analysis of the annular size is relevant to prosthetic valve sizing (**Fig. 1**), and understanding the degree and pattern of calcification in the annulus is important concerning procedural technique (**Fig. 2**).[10] Vitally important is the understanding of the remaining LVOT created by the boundaries of the new valve prosthesis/anterior mitral leaflet and the septum, or neo-LVOT; this is discussed in greater detail later. Inadequate space in the neo-LVOT is among the most common reasons for the exclusion of patients for the current TMVR device trials or ViV/ViR/ valve-in-MAC (ViMAC). For

those patients undergoing transapical access TMVR, the left ventricular (LV) puncture site target is also chosen based on the most coaxial approach to the mitral valve plane.

The preoperative assessment of neo-LVOT post-TMVR is crucial. This assessment can be performed by careful evaluation of the preprocedural three-dimensional cardiac gated computed tomography scan.[11,12] Multiphase and explicitly early systolic evaluation of the neo-LVOT area is preferred, with an eye toward the narrowest possible dimension.[12,13] This area is measured using a double oblique method by identifying the basalmost insertion points of the mitral leaflets and implanting a virtual valve (typically 20% atrial and 80% ventricular). A neo-LVOT area of less than or equal to 189.4 mm^2 has a sensitivity of 100% and a specificity of 96.8% for foretelling post-TMVR LVOT obstruction.[14] Another study suggested a cutoff of 1.7 cm^2 (sensitivity 96.2% and specificity 92.3%).[15] In addition to the neo-LVOT area, aortomitral angulation closer to 90° and a small left ventricle size are independent predictors of post-TMVR LVOT obstruction.[16]

VALVE IN VALVE/VALVE IN RING/VALVE IN MITRAL ANNULAR CALCIFICATION

ViV/ViR/ViMAC can be performed using the balloon-expandable Edwards SAPIEN 3 TAVR system. The mitral ViV application is extremely helpful for preoperative planning and device choice and is widely available across iPhone and android phone app stores. These procedures are mostly performed antegrade across the interatrial septum. Recently, the contemporary experience with SAPIEN 3 valve for transcatheter mitral ViV replacement was published.[17] The study comprised more than 1500 patients and the procedural success rate was nearly 97%. The 1-year mortality postintervention was nearly 17% and, not surprisingly, the mortality was substantially higher with transapical access compared with transeptal access. Postintervention there was sustained improvement in heart failure symptoms, with an average mitral mean gradient of 7 mm Hg at 1 year.[17]

A global multicenter registry of 116 patients reported a 30-day mortality of 25% and 1-year mortality of 53.7% post-TMVR with balloon-expandable aortic valves in patients with MAC.[18] A systematic review and meta-analysis of 4 studies compared periprocedural outcomes between ViMAC and ViV/ViR cohorts.[19] The periprocedural mortality was higher (ViMAC 31% vs ViV/ViR 7%) and was associated with inferior procedural success rates (ViMAC 64% vs ViV/ViR

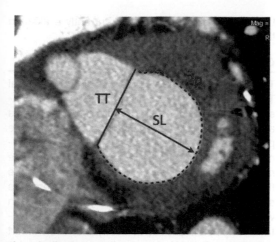

Fig. 1. Mitral annulus measurement using multidetector computed tomography. SL, septal-to-lateral distance; TT, trigone-to-trigone distance; 2p, perimeter. (*From* Faggioni L, Gabelloni M, Accogli S, Angelillis M, Costa G, Spontoni P, et al. Preprocedural planning of transcatheter mitral valve interventions by multidetector CT: What the radiologist needs to know. Eur J Radiol Open. 2018;5:131-40.)

91%) in the ViMAC cohort compared with ViV/ViR cohort.[19] The ViMAC cohort had a higher risk of LVOT obstruction (ViMAC 36% vs ViV/ViR 4%) and surgical conversion (ViMAC 9% vs ViV/ViR 2%) compared with ViV/ViR cohorts.[19] In addition, ViMAC procedures are associated with hemolytic anemia, which can range from mild to transfusion dependent and sometimes is complicated by pigment-induced nephropathy; this is likely

caused by paravalvular regurgitation with inadequate annular sealing.[20] The incidence of second valve implantation has been reported to be higher in ViR patients (12.1%) compared with ViMAC (5.2%) and ViV patients (2.5%).[21] ViR cohorts also have a higher risk of greater than or equal to moderate residual MR (ViR 18.4% vs ViMAC 13.8% vs ViV 5.6%) and often require paravalvular leak closure (ViR 7.8% vs ViMAC 0.0% vs ViV 2.2%).

More recently, a combined approach to ViR and ViMAC procedures using laceration of the anterior mitral valve leaflet to prevent LVOT obstruction (LAMPOON) and/or alcohol septal ablation (ASA) to prevent LVOT obstruction has been used. This approach was studied in a cohort of 40 patients that included 28 ViMAC and 12 ViR patients.[22] Using this algorithm, 16 patients underwent LAMPOON and 3 patients underwent ASA before TMVR. The 30-day mortality was 15%, valve embolization or late migration was seen in 5 patients, and technical success was seen in 63% of the patients.[22]

In summary, the literature available thus far strongly supports the role of transcatheter mitral ViV in degenerated bioprosthetic valves. The mortality and complications are higher in patients undergoing transcatheter mitral ViR and ViMAC procedures.[15,18,21,23,24] ViR/ViMAC are more often complicated by paravalvular regurgitation necessitating closure compared with the ViV procedures.[15,18,21,23–28] Further, these patients also show a higher rate of LVOT obstruction and consideration should be given to preemptive

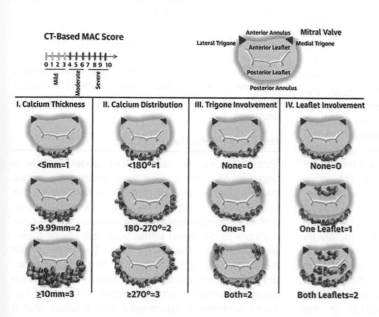

Fig. 2. Multidetector computed tomography scoring system for MAC. (*From* Guerrero M, Wang DD, Pursnani A, Eleid M, Khalique O, Urena M, et al. A Cardiac Computed Tomography-Based Score to Categorize Mitral Annular Calcification Severity and Predict Valve Embolization. JACC Cardiovascular imaging. 2020;13(9):1945-57.)

LAMPOON and/or ASA to mitigate this risk.[15,18,19,21,23,24]

NATIVE VALVE TRANSCATHETER MITRAL VALVE REPLACEMENT DEVICES

There are several valves currently being assessed in clinical trials, although most of the data are limited with regard to the number of patients treated and have been presented at conferences but not yet published in peer-reviewed journals. Therefore, a detailed analysis is not possible, but a summary of the devices and results thus far is provided herein (**Fig. 3**, **Tables 1** and **2**).

AltaValve

AltaValve system (4C Medical) is a 32-Fr supra-annular system with a self-expanding spherical nitinol frame that consists of a 27-mm bovine pericardial valve.[29] This valve can be delivered trans-apically as well as transeptally.[29,30] The first AltaValve implanted via a transapical approach was performed successfully with regard to valve positioning and deployment; however, the procedure was complicated by significant LV bleeding.[29] The patient passed away 5 days later.[29] The procedure performed via the transeptal route was successful in a 77-year-old man who was discharged 9 days later. The patient had good mitral valve function and no LVOT gradient.[30] The supra-annular position of this valve is helpful to minimize LVOT obstruction and prevent valve embolization/migration. The AltaValve early feasibility study is currently underway (NCT03997305).

Cardiovalve (Cardiovalve)

Cardiovalve is a self-expanding platform with a bovine pericardial trileaflet valve with atrial and ventricular frames that is, available in 3 sizes (M, L, XL). This valve is delivered using a 28-Fr transfemoral sheath and is deployed in 3 phases. Initially the mitral leaflets are grasped, followed by the deployment of the atrial flanges, and lastly the final deployment of the valve. This valve is inspired by the surgical mitral prostheses that are designed to provide a low ventricular profile and reduce the risk of LVOT obstruction, with good durability. This valve has been assessed in 5 patients so far with promising procedural results, with 100% implantation rate and 80% of patients had complete resolution of MR. The 30-day mortality was 60%, mostly as a result of access site complications. The AHEAD (European Feasibility Study of High Surgical Risk Patients With Severe MR Treated With the Cardiovalve Transfemoral Mitral Valve System Study) studies (NCT03813524, NCT03339115) in the United States and Europe are currently evaluating the feasibility of the Cardiovalve.

Cephea (Abbott Vascular)

The Cephea valve is a self-expanding transseptal TMVR system with a double-disk design that consists of an outer ring that conforms to the annulus and an inner ring that consists of a trileaflet bovine pericardial valve. They are available in 32-mm, 36-mm, and 40-mm sizes. This system anchors the mitral annulus by axial compression. In 2019, the first-in-human implant of the Cephea system was successfully performed in an 83-year-old woman with degenerative MR.[31] Six months after implantation she had improved clinically (New York Heart Association [NYHA] class I) with good mitral valve function (mean gradient 3 mm Hg), no paravalvular leak, and no LVOT gradient.[31] Further trials are needed to evaluate the safety and feasibility of the device and are underway (NCT03988946).

EVOQUE (Edwards Lifesciences)

EVOQUE is a transseptal nitinol self-expanding system with a bovine pericardial valve. The ventricular segment has 9 anchors that attach to the mitral valve leaflets and chords. The atrial segment has a sealing skirt to prevent paravalvular leak. The device can be delivered via a 28-Fr transfemoral sheath and is available in 2 dimensions (44 and 48 mm). The three-dimensional delivery system allows precise manipulation and tilted deployment of the device at the mitral annulus. The rationale behind the tilted deployment of the device is to reduce the risk of LVOT obstruction. The early experience in 14 patients with moderate to severe MR showed a technical success rate of 92.9%.[32] One patient needed open heart surgery and 2 patients had strokes.[32] Two individuals needed paravalvular leak closure and 1 of them underwent ASA.[32] A reduction to NYHA functional class II was seen in 82% of the individuals. NCT02718001 is an early feasibility study that is currently in progress.

HighLife (HighLife Medical)

This TMVR system uses a ViR model. Initially, a ring (32–48 mm) is deployed across the mitral valve (subannular) in a retrograde fashion via the transfemoral artery. Following this, a 28-mm self-expanding trileaflet valve made of bovine pericardium is deployed either transapically or transseptally inside the mitral ring. This ViR model hypothetically reduces the risk of LVOT obstruction and paravalvular leak. Initial results have been presented among 15 patients. Thirteen patients underwent successful implantation and 2

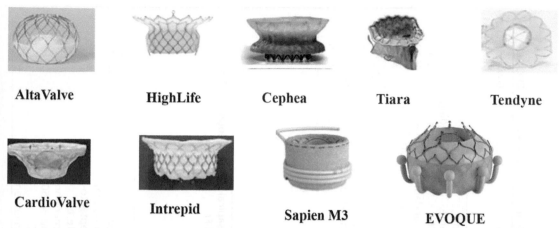

AltaValve   **HighLife**   **Cephea**   **Tiara**   **Tendyne**

CardioValve   **Intrepid**   **Sapien M3**   **EVOQUE**

Fig. 3. TMVR devices in evaluation.

patients needed open heart surgery. The 1-month mortality was 20%. An early feasibility trial (NCT02974881) is recruiting patients to assess this system.

SAPIEN M3 (Edwards Lifesciences)

The M3 system is another device that follows the ViR concept. Unlike the HighLIfe system, the ring (nitinol dock) is delivered across the atrial septum and deployed in the mitral valve apparatus. The valve is like the SAPIEN S3 and has a knitted poly-ethylene terephthalate skirt to achieve a tight seal. The initial feasibility study consisting of 35 patients was promising, with a technical success of 88.6% and an all-cause mortality of 2.9%.[33,34] The Encircle trial of this device is in its initial stages (NCT03230747).

Intrepid (Medtronic Inc)

The Intrepid is a transapical, self-expanding, nitinol valve and consists of a dual-stent conformable symmetric model that does not need a rotational align-ment. The outer stent frame conforms to the mitral annulus, whereas the inner stent consists of a trileaf-let 27-mm valve made from bovine pericardium. The valve anchors to the mitral annulus, left ventricle, with perimeter oversizing, and is delivered using a retrievable 35-Fr transapical system. The early experience with this device in a prospective study consisting of 50 patients at high or extreme risk for conventional mitral valve replacement is feasible. The mean age of the cohort was 73 years, with pre-dominantly secondary MR (84%). The average Soci-ety for Thoracic Surgery score of the cohort was 6.4%. The procedural success rate of the device was 96%. The 1-month mortality was 14%, and there was a substantial improvement in functional status and Minnesota Heart Failure Questionnaire

scores.[35] The APOLLO TMVR trial (TMVR With the Medtronic Intrepid TMVR System in Patients With Severe Symptomatic Mitral Regurgitation; NCT03242642) is currently enrolling patients with moderate to severe or severe symptomatic MR and will compare TMVR with conventional mitral valve replacement.

Tendyne (Abbott Vascular)

The Tendyne TMVR system is another transapical system that is a fully retrievable and repositionable device, and currently has the largest clinical expe-rience worldwide, with more than 400 valves implanted. This 34-Fr system delivers 2 self-expanding nitinol stents and a trileaflet porcine pericardial valve. It also consists of an apical pad that anchors the valve to the LV apex. This device has gained the CE (Conformité Européenne) mark in Europe.[36,37]

The Global Feasibility Study had a sample size of 100 individuals with primary or secondary MR who had a mean age of more than 75 years. The cohort had a mean Society of Thoracic Surgeons (STS) score of 7.8 and the technical success rate was 96%. The 30-day mortality was 6% and 1-year survival postprocedure was 72%. At 1 year, more than 88% of the individuals who survived had substantial improvements in 6-minute walk distance and quality of life.[37]

This device has been also studied in individuals with severe MAC and MR.[36] There was complete resolution of MR in 9 patients who had a survival rate of 78% at 1 year.[36] The SUMMIT trial (Clinical Trial to Evaluate the Safety and Effectiveness of Using the Tendyne Mitral Valve System for the Treatment of Symptomatic Mitral Regurgitation; NCT03433274) consists of a randomized study, nonrandomized study, and an MAC registry. The

Table 1
Summary of all the transcatheter mitral valve replacement devices and future feasibility studies

Device	AltaValve	Cardiovalve	HighLife	Intrepid	Tiara	SAPIEN M3	Tendyne	Cephea	EVOQUE
Manufacturer	4C Medical Technologies	Cardiovalve	HighLife SAS	Medtronic	Neovasc	Edwards Lifesciences	Abbott	Abbott	Edwards Lifesciences
Design	Self-expanding, nitinol	NA	Self-expanding, nitinol	Double stent, self-expanding, nitinol	Self-expanding, nitinol	Balloon-expandable, cobalt-chromium frame	Double frame, self-expandable, nitinol	A self-expanding system with a double-disk design	Self-expanding, nitinol
Leaflets	Trileaflet bovine	NA	Trileaflet bovine	Trileaflet bovine	Trileaflet bovine	Trileaflet bovine	Trileaflet porcine	NA	Trileaflet porcine
Anchoring mechanism	Spherical frame shape	NA	Valve in subannular mitral ring; external anchor	Radial force and small cleats on the outer stent engage leaflets	3 ventricular anchoring tabs (on the fibrous trigone and posterior shelf of the annulus)	Nitinol dock system	Apical tether	Mitral annulus double disk	Mitral annulus leaflets/annulus
Access site	Transapical 32 Fr	Transfemoral-transseptal 28 Fr	Transapical (transfemoral artery for loop placement) 39 Fr	Transapical 35 Fr	Transapical 32 Fr (35-mm valve) 36 Fr (40-mm valve)	Transfemoral 20 Fr	Transapical 34 Fr	Transseptal	Transseptal 28 Fr
Valve dimensions	27 mm	3 sizes (M, L, XL)	31	27 (with 3 outer stent sizes: 43, 46, and 50 mm)	35 and 40 mm	29 mm	Outer frame 30–43 mm (septal-to-lateral dimension) and 34–50 (IC dimension)	Sizes 32, 36, and 40 mm	44 and 48 mm

Recapturable	Partial	Partial	No	Yes	No	Partial	Yes	Yes	No
Trial	NCT03997305	AHEAD studies NCT03813524, NCT03339115	NCT02974881	APOLLO TMVR trial NCT03242642	TIARA-I (NCT02276547) and TIARA-II (NCT03039855)	NCT03230747	The SUMMIT study (NCT03433274)	NCT03988946	NCT02718001

Abbreviation: IC, intercommissural; NA, not available.

Table 2
Summary of the early data with upcoming transcatheter mitral valve replacement devices

Valve	Intrepid	Tendyne	EVOQUE	SAPIEN M3	Cardiovalve	HighLife	AltaValve	Tiara	Cephea
Publication Year	2018	2019	2020	2019	2020	2018	2019	2020	2019
Patients Enrolled	50	100	14	15	5	15	2	79	1
Procedural Success (%)	98	96	93	89	100	87	100	92	100
Follow-up (d)	173	416.7	30	30	30	30	9	30	196
Residual MR $\geq$ +2 (%)	0	0	0	2	0	0	0	3	0
Mortality (%)	22	26	7	2	60	21	50	12.3	0

patients in the randomized trial will be randomized to Tendyne or a MitraClip system.

Tiara (NeoVasc Inc)

Tiara has an asymmetric D-shaped design and is composed of a self-expanding nitinol frame, 2 axial anchors (anterior and posterior), and a trileaflet bovine pericardial valve. This device reduces LVOT obstruction because the anterior tab grabs the anterior mitral leaflet and because of its

D-shaped design. This transapical device is available in 2 dimensions: 35 mm (32 Fr) and 40 mm (36 Fr). A transeptal delivery system is currently being developed. Feasibility studies TIARA-I (NCT02276547) and TIARA-II (NCT03039855) are yet to be officially published. The procedural success rate was more than 90%, but more than 10% of the patients needed surgical reintervention. The 30-day mortality was 12.3%, with a device migration rate of 7%. None of the patients

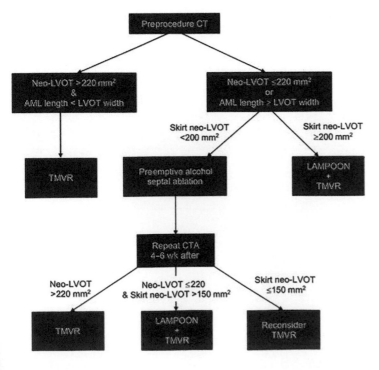

Fig. 4. Algorithmic approach for TMVR. AML, anterior mitral leaflet; CTA, computed tomography angiography. (*From* Tiwana J, Aldea G, Levin DB, Johnson K, Don CW, Dvir D, et al. Contemporary Transcatheter Mitral Valve Replacement for Mitral Annular Calcification or Ring. JACC Cardiovascular interventions. 2020;13(20):2388-98.)

developed LVOT obstruction and, at discharge, 88% of the patients had no or trivial MR.

MITIGATION STRATEGIES TO PREVENT LEFT VENTRICULAR OUTFLOW TRACT OBSTRUCTION

TMVR in ViV procedures, ViR, and MAC is possible; however, these patients are prone to develop severe LVOT obstruction resulting in hemodynamic compromise.[18] The rates of LVOT obstruction resulting in hemodynamic compromise post-TMVR in individuals with MAC are as high as 11%, and the mortality for these patients is substantial.[18,38] Over time, investigators have used several different strategies to circumvent this issue.

Alcohol Septal Ablation

ASA was used as a bailout strategy initially and more recently has been implemented as a preemptive strategy.[22,24,39,40] In the early report of using ASA as a bailout strategy, only 4 of the 6 patients survived post-TMVR.[24] The first-in-human study of 30 patients evaluating ASA as a preemptive strategy before TMVR was recently published.[40] Baseline imaging revealed a median end-diastolic LV septal thickness of 13.5 mm, median baseline neo-LVOT surface area before ASA of 85.1 mm^2, and a baseline median peak LVOT gradient of 5.5 mm Hg.[40] A median increase in the neo-LVOT area by 111.2 mm^2 was observed ($P<.0001$) after a median duration of 40 days post-ASA.[40] Eight patients experienced clinical improvement after ASA and no longer had an indication for TMVR, and 2 patients died after ASA but before TMVR.[40] The pacemaker implantation rate was 16.7%. More encouragingly, this publication reported post-TMVR 30-day mortality of 5.3%, with a TMVR success rate of 100%.[40]

LAMPOON

The LAMPOON procedure was devised to prevent LVOT obstruction. LAMPOON is a catheter-based electrosurgical procedure where the anterior leaflet is lacerated before deployment of the mitral valve. The laceration of the A2 leaflet is performed by first using a 0.36-mm (0.014-inch) stiff guidewire (Astato XS 20, Asahi-Intecc, Nagoya, Japan) to anterogradely puncture the base of the A2 mitral valve scallop via a 145-cm Piggyback Wire Converter (Vascular Solutions, Minneapolis, MN) that has a 0.89-mm (0.035-inch) polymer jacket and provides electrical insulation. The wire is then snared via the ventricle and the leaflet is lacerated from base to tip. In the feasibility study of 30

patients, 30-day survival was 93% with no strokes.[40,41]

In addition to the procedural technique discussed earlier, it is possible in patients with a mitral ring or bioprosthetic to avoid the initial leaflet perforation altogether and instead use the tip-to-base technique.[41–43] For this procedure, the wire is passed antegrade through the mitral valve and snared via a retrograde catheter. The cutting surface is then electrified and pulled from tip to base, and the heart is shielded from further injury by the prosthetic annulus. **Fig. 4** shows the role of a hybrid algorithm in ViMAC/ViR procedures that has a success rate of 63%.[22]

POST–TRANSCATHETER MITRAL VALVE REPLACEMENT ATRIAL SEPTAL CLOSURE

The role of iatrogenic atrial septal closure is controversial post-TMVR.[44] This decision depends on the left atrial, ventricular pressures as well as on the degree of right ventricular failure and volume status. The atrial septum is often closed for the spontaneous right-to-left shunt and/or hypoxia most commonly seen in the presence of severe pulmonary hypertension, right ventricular dysfunction, or concomitant severe tricuspid regurgitation.[44] The MITHRAS trial was a clinical trial that included 80 patients with Qp/Qs of greater than or equal to 1.3 post-TMVR and randomized them to closure using the Occlutech ASD occluder or conservative management at 1-month post-TMVR.[45] Baseline clinical and echocardiographic features were similar across the 2 cohorts. There was no difference in mortality and rehospitalization post-TMVR across the 2 cohorts. The trial was underpowered to assess for differences in special subgroups such as a large defect with spontaneous shunts and the degree of right ventricular failure.[45]

SUMMARY

The future of TMVR seems promising, although the progress in TMVR device technology has been slow. The current evidence is robust for the use of balloon-expandable valves in degenerated bioprosthetic valves. ViR and ViMAC procedures are far more complicated and have inferior outcomes but may present as the only available options for many patients. TMVR for native mitral valve regurgitation is currently reserved for patients with poor anatomy for transcatheter mitral valve repair using the US Food and Drug Administration–approved MitraClip edge-to-edge repair. There are many different transapically and transfemorally delivered TMVR devices in various stages of clinical trials for native valve disease, primary MR. Most of these trials show excellent procedural success, although further study is needed to establish valve durability and longer-term patient outcomes, and to better understand patient selection.

CLINICS CARE POINTS

- The mitral valve annulus is a dynamic, saddle-shaped structure that is supported by a complex subvalvular apparatus. Wide variations in pathophysiology are seen, including but not limited to MAC, functional MR, primary MR, MS, and mixed mitral valve disease.

- Echocardiographic features favoring TMVR rather than transcatheter mitral valve repair include MR origins that are broad along the coaptation line, large coaptation gap, mitral valve area less than 3.5 cm², multiple prolapsing segments, mixed mitral valve disease with predominant MS, severe calcification at the grasping zone, short (<7 mm) and significantly tethered posterior mitral valve leaflet, and a cleft or perforation.

- Cardiac computed tomography is an extremely important tool for preprocedural planning in native TMVR as well as ViV, ViR, and ViMAC procedures to understand the annulus, neo-LVOT dimensions, fluoroscopic angles for valve implantation, and access site assessment.

- Transcatheter mitral ViV is a safe and effective procedure for most patients with a degenerated bioprosthetic valve. In contrast, the outcomes of transcatheter mitral ViR/ViMAC are suboptimal and these procedures are generally reserved for patients at high or extreme surgical risk.

- Intentional laceration of the anterior mitral leaflet and ASA may be effective mitigation strategies in appropriately selected patients to avoid LVOT obstruction in high-risk anatomies of ViR and ViMAC.

- Many devices are currently under investigation, and the ideal device is yet to be established for native TMVR.

ACKNOWLEDGMENTS

Nil.

DISCLOSURES

The authors have no relationships with industry.

REFERENCES

1. Mack MJ, Leon MB, Thourani VH, et al. Transcatheter aortic-valve replacement with a balloon-expandable valve in low-risk patients. N Engl J Med 2019;380(18):1695–705.

2. Popma JJ, Deeb GM, Yakubov SJ, et al. Transcatheter aortic-valve replacement with a self-expanding valve in low-risk patients. N Engl J Med 2019; 380(18):1706–15.

3. Messika-Zeitoun D, Iung B, Armoiry X, et al. Impact of mitral regurgitation severity and left ventricular remodeling on outcome after mitraclip implantation: results from the mitra-FR trial. JACC Cardiovasc Imaging 2020;S1936-878X(20):30645–8. https://doi.org/10.1016/j.jcmg.2020.07.021.

4. Asmarats L, Puri R, Latib A, et al. Transcatheter tricuspid valve interventions: landscape, challenges, and future directions. J Am Coll Cardiol 2018;71(25):2935–56.

5. Holzer RJ, Hijazi ZM. Transcatheter pulmonary valve replacement: state of the art. Catheter Cardiovasc Interv 2016;87(1):117–28.

6. Feldman T, Foster E, Glower DD, et al. Percutaneous repair or surgery for mitral regurgitation. N Engl J Med 2011;364(15):1395–406.

7. Stone GW, Lindenfeld J, Abraham WT, et al. Transcatheter mitral-valve repair in patients with heart failure. N Engl J Med 2018;379(24):2307–18.

8. Mackensen GB, Lee JC, Wang DD, et al. Role of echocardiography in transcatheter mitral valve replacement in native mitral valves and mitral rings. J Am Soc Echocardiogr 2018;31(4):475–90.

9. Natarajan N, Patel P, Bartel T, et al. Peri-procedural imaging for transcatheter mitral valve replacement. Cardiovasc Diagn Ther 2016;6(2):144–59.

10. Guerrero M, Wang DD, Pursnani A, et al. A cardiac computed tomography-based score to categorize mitral annular calcification severity and predict valve embolization. JACC Cardiovasc Imaging 2020; 13(9):1945–57.

11. Alharbi Y, Otton J, Muller DWM, et al. Predicting the outcome of transcatheter mitral valve implantation using image-based computational models. J Cardiovasc Comput Tomogr 2020;14(4): 335–42.

12. Meduri CU, Reardon MJ, Lim DS, et al. Novel multiphase assessment for predicting left ventricular outflow tract obstruction before transcatheter mitral valve replacement. JACC Cardiovasc Interv 2019; 12(23):2402–12.

13. Lisko J, Kamioka N, Gleason P, et al. Prevention and treatment of left ventricular outflow tract obstruction after transcatheter mitral valve replacement. Interv Cardiol Clin 2019;8(3):279–85.

14. Wang DD, Eng MH, Greenbaum AB, et al. Validating a prediction modeling tool for left ventricular outflow

tract (LVOT) obstruction after transcatheter mitral valve replacement (TMVR). Catheter Cardiovasc Interv 2018;92(2):379–87.

15. Yoon SH, Bleiziffer S, Latib A, et al. Predictors of left ventricular outflow tract obstruction after transcatheter mitral valve replacement. JACC Cardiovasc Interv 2019;12(2):182–93.

16. Blanke P, Naoum C, Webb J, et al. Multimodality imaging in the context of transcatheter mitral valve replacement: establishing consensus among modalities and disciplines. JACC Cardiovasc Imaging 2015;8(10):1191–208.

17. Whisenant B, Kapadia SR, Eleid MF, et al. One-year outcomes of mitral valve-in-valve using the SAPIEN 3 transcatheter heart valve. JAMA Cardiol 2020;5(11):1245–52.

18. Guerrero M, Urena M, Himbert D, et al. 1-year outcomes of transcatheter mitral valve replacement in patients with severe mitral annular calcification. J Am Coll Cardiol 2018;71(17):1841–53.

19. Ribeiro RVP, Yanagawa B, Légaré JF, et al. Clinical outcomes of mitral valve intervention in patients with mitral annular calcification: a systematic review and meta-analysis. J Card Surg 2020;35(1):66–74.

20. El-Sabawi B, Guerrero M, Eleid M, et al. TCT CONNECT-340 hemolysis after transcatheter mitral valve replacement: incidence, patient characteristics, and clinical outcomes. J Am Coll Cardiol 2020;76(17 Supplement S):B146–7.

21. Yoon SH, Whisenant BK, Bleiziffer S, et al. Outcomes of transcatheter mitral valve replacement for degenerated bioprostheses, failed annuloplasty rings, and mitral annular calcification. Eur Heart J 2019;40(5):441–51.

22. Tiwana J, Aldea G, Levin DB, et al. Contemporary transcatheter mitral valve replacement for mitral annular calcification or ring. JACC Cardiovasc Interv 2020;13(20):2388–98.

23. Babaliaros VC, Greenbaum AB, Khan JM, et al. Intentional percutaneous laceration of the anterior mitral leaflet to prevent outflow obstruction during transcatheter mitral valve replacement: first-in-human experience. JACC Cardiovasc Interv 2017;10(8):798–809.

24. Guerrero M, Wang DD, Himbert D, et al. Short-term results of alcohol septal ablation as a bail-out strategy to treat severe left ventricular outflow tract obstruction after transcatheter mitral valve replacement in patients with severe mitral annular calcification. Catheter Cardiovasc Interv 2017;90(7):1220–6.

25. Eleid MF, Whisenant BK, Cabalka AK, et al. Early outcomes of percutaneous transvenous transseptal transcatheter valve implantation in failed bioprosthetic mitral valves, ring annuloplasty, and severe mitral annular calcification. JACC Cardiovasc Interv 2017;10(19):1932–42.

26. Yoon SH, Whisenant BK, Bleiziffer S, et al. Transcatheter mitral valve replacement for degenerated bioprosthetic valves and failed annuloplasty rings. J Am Coll Cardiol 2017;70(9):1121–31.

27. Ye J, Cheung A, Yamashita M, et al. Transcatheter aortic and mitral valve-in-valve implantation for failed surgical bioprosthetic valves: an 8-year single-center experience. JACC Cardiovasc Interv 2015;8(13):1735–44.

28. Bouleti C, Fassa AA, Himbert D, et al. Transfemoral implantation of transcatheter heart valves after deterioration of mitral bioprosthesis or previous ring annuloplasty. JACC Cardiovasc Interv 2015;8(1 Pt A):83–91.

29. Goel SS, Zuck V, Christy J, et al. Transcatheter mitral valve therapy with novel Supra-Annular AltaValve: first experience in the United States. JACC Case Rep 2019;1(5):761–4.

30. Ferreira-Neto AN, Dagenais F, Bernier M, et al. Transcatheter mitral valve replacement with a new supra-annular valve. JACC Cardiovasc Interv 2019;12(2):208–9.

31. Modine T, Vahl TP, Khalique OK, et al. First-in-human implant of the cephea transseptal mitral valve replacement system. Circ Cardiovasc Interv 2019;12(9):e008003.

32. Webb J, Hensey M, Fam N, et al. Transcatheter mitral valve replacement with the transseptal EVOQUE system. JACC Cardiovasc Interv 2020;13(20):2418–26.

33. Webb JG, Murdoch DJ, Boone RH, et al. Percutaneous transcatheter mitral valve replacement: first-in-human experience with a new transseptal system. J Am Coll Cardiol 2019;73(11):1239–46.

34. Makkar R, O'Neill W, Whisenant B, et al. TCT-8 updated 30-day outcomes for the U.S. early feasibility study of the SAPIEN M3 transcatheter mitral valve replacement system. J Am Coll Cardiol 2019;74(13_Supplement):B8-B.

35. Bapat V, Rajagopal V, Meduri C, et al. Early experience with new transcatheter mitral valve replacement. J Am Coll Cardiol 2018;71(1):12–21.

36. Sorajja P, Gössl M, Babaliaros V, et al. Novel transcatheter mitral valve prosthesis for patients with severe mitral annular calcification. J Am Coll Cardiol 2019;74(11):1431–40.

37. Sorajja P, Moat N, Badhwar V, et al. Initial feasibility study of a new transcatheter mitral prosthesis: the first 100 patients. J Am Coll Cardiol 2019;73(11):1250–60.

38. Khan JM, Rogers T, Schenke WH, et al. Intentional laceration of the anterior mitral valve leaflet to prevent left ventricular outflow tract obstruction during transcatheter mitral valve replacement: pre-clinical findings. JACC Cardiovasc Interv 2016;9(17):1835–43.

39. Long A, Mahoney P. Sequential use of alcohol septal ablation and electrosurgical leaflet resection prior to

transcatheter mitral valve replacement. J Invasive Cardiol 2020;32(2):E36–41.

40. Wang DD, Guerrero M, Eng MH, et al. Alcohol septal ablation to prevent left ventricular outflow tract obstruction during transcatheter mitral valve replacement: first-in-man study. JACC Cardiovasc Interv 2019;12(13):1268–79.

41. Khan JM, Babaliaros VC, Greenbaum AB, et al. Anterior leaflet laceration to prevent ventricular outflow tract obstruction during transcatheter mitral valve replacement. J Am Coll Cardiol 2019;73(20): 2521–34.

42. Case BC, Khan JM, Satler LF, et al. Tip-to-base LAMPOON to prevent left ventricular outflow tract

obstruction in valve-in-valve transcatheter mitral valve replacement. JACC Cardiovasc Interv 2020; 13(9):1126–8.

43. Khan JM, Rogers T, Greenbaum AB, et al. Transcatheter electrosurgery: JACC state-of-the-art review. J Am Coll Cardiol 2020;75(12):1455–70.

44. Beri N, Singh GD, Smith TW, et al. Iatrogenic atrial septal defect closure after transseptal mitral valve interventions: indications and outcomes. Catheter Cardiovasc Interv 2019;94(6):829–36.

45. Lurz P, Unterhuber M, Rommel K-P, et al. Closure of iatrogenic atrial septal defect following transcatheter mitral valve repair: the randomized MITHRAS trial. Circulation 2021;143(3):292–4.

Echocardiographic Evaluation of Successful Mitral Valve Repair or Need for a Second Pump Run in the Operating Room

Mitsuhiko Ota, MD[a],*, Takeshi Kitai, MD, PhD[b]

KEYWORDS

- Mitral regurgitation
- Mitral valve repair
- Intraoperative transesophageal echocardiography

KEY POINTS

- Intraoperative transesophageal echocardiography provides immediate diagnostic feedback and assessment of results during valve repair procedures and has become an essential guiding tool for decision-making among surgeons.
- Systematic echocardiographic evaluation of mitral valve repair based on a specific algorithm is mandatory.
- Three-dimensional transesophageal echocardiography plays a pivotal role in both preprocedural and postprocedural assessments in mitral valve repair.

INTRODUCTION

Mitral valve (MV) repair has become the gold standard surgical procedure for significant mitral regurgitation (MR).[1] The objectives of MV repair are to preserve or restore full leaflet motion, to create a good surface for leaflet coaptation, and to remodel and stabilize the entire annulus.

Detailed preoperative echocardiographic assessment of the MV apparatus is crucial for surgical planning.[2] Three-dimensional (3D) transesophageal echocardiography (TEE) plays a pivotal role in both preprocedural and postprocedural assessments in MV repair and has become widely adopted in echocardiographic laboratories and operating rooms worldwide.[3–6] In the operating room, intraoperative

TEE evaluation requires accurate analysis of the MV anatomy and details of affected valve lesions.[7] Furthermore, as surgeons must rapidly decide whether cardiopulmonary bypass (CPB) should be continued to be weaning off or a second pump run should be selected, the echocardiographer conducting intraoperative TEE is required to be trained according to a certain algorithm. In particular, when the saline test results are difficult to judge the extent of residual regurgitation, evaluation by intraoperative TEE may be faster and more accurate under physiologic cardiac movement after weaning off the CPB.

The present review aimed to examine the current clinical role of intraoperative TEE in MV repair in the operating room.

Funding sources: None.
Declarations of interest: None.
[a] Department of Cardiovascular Center, Toranomon Hospital, 2-2-2 Toranomon, Minato-ku, Tokyo 105-8470, Japan; [b] Department of Cardiovascular Medicine, Kobe City Medical Center General Hospital, 2-1-1 Minatojima Minamimachi, Chuo-ku, Kobe 650-0047, Japan
* Corresponding author.
E-mail address: mohta5288923@gmail.com

ROLE OF INTRAOPERATIVE TRANSESOPHAGEAL ECHOCARDIOGRAPHY IN MITRAL VALVE REPAIR: WHAT IS SUCCESSFUL MITRAL VALVE REPAIR?

Echocardiographic imaging of the MV before and immediately after repair is crucial for immediate and long-term outcomes.[8–10] Postrepair echocardiographic imaging reveals the new baseline anatomy, assesses the function, and determines whether further intervention is required.

Successful MV repair is defined as a decrease in MR severity to mild or less without mitral stenosis or left ventricular outflow tract obstruction owing to systolic anterior motion (SAM). The surgeon should achieve complete MR elimination while minimizing valve area reduction.[11] An inadequate technique may result in either residual MR or mitral stenosis, which can be shown using intraoperative TEE. Such information will improve treatment options, enhance the timing of invasive therapies, and lead to advancements in repair techniques, thereby yielding better outcomes.

Quantitatively, an ideal MV repair should restore competency (MR <1+), ensure adequate patency (mean gradient of ≤ 6 mm Hg and MV area of ≤ 1.5 cm^2), and have durability (>10 years without significant MR and/or reoperation).[12–16] Because intraoperative TEE provides immediate diagnostic feedback and assessment of results during valve repair procedures, it has become an essential guiding tool for decision-making among surgeons.[11]

In the operating room, optimizing the communication between the surgeon and the cardiologist performing echocardiography is mandatory to ensure the best possible outcomes for patients. Because postprocedural echocardiographic evaluation can be conducted immediately after aortic cross-clamp release, the cardiologist must be on standby in the operating room before the completion of left atrial suture. Furthermore, obtaining information from the surgeon on how valve repair was performed is important. An online environment in which the surgical field can be viewed from all medical record terminals in the hospital enables cardiologists to observe directly the repaired valve remotely from an echocardiographic laboratory (**Fig. 1**). The key to successful MV repair is that the final 3D images of the repaired valve can be shared simultaneously between surgeons and cardiologist when the CPB was weaned off.

Because the procedures used in MV repair differ depending on the facility and surgeon, it is necessary to share information among echocardiographers on surgical techniques that are often used in daily clinical practice.

Systematic echocardiographic evaluation of MV repair is mandatory. At the initial time when the CPB is weaned off, the most sufficient imaging view for the evaluation of the repaired MV is the midesophageal (ME) long axis (LAX) view, not the 4-chamber view or mitral commissural view. The reasons for this are as follows: (1) it is easy to observe the dynamic state of the aortic valve starting to open, because the volume is loaded to the left ventricle. (2) Both the anterior and posterior MV leaflets can be visualized simultaneously. (3) The mobility, coaptation, and regurgitation of the repaired MV, as well as the iatrogenic regurgitation of the aortic valve, can be evaluated at a glance. The following checkpoints for the assessment of MV repair are recommended (**Fig. 2**).

Checkpoint 1: Residual Mitral Regurgitation

A successfully repaired MV should not have more than mild MR immediately after separation from the CPB.[17,18] The principles for the echocardiographic assessment of residual MR are the same as those for the evaluation of the native valve.[13] Such assessment should be performed with a sufficiently loaded left ventricle and a systolic blood pressure of greater than 100 mm Hg to simulate physiologic status and avoid residual MR underestimation. Surgeons need to put up a few minutes for proper volume and afterload settings and for their echocardiographic assessments, which results in the best benefit to patients. MR jet area with color flow Doppler (CFD) is the most common method used for the rapid quantitative evaluation of residual MR.

If residual MR is more than mild or occurs in eccentric jets, a detailed assessment is required to determine the mechanism of residual MR and aid in the revision of re-repair on a second CPB pump run (second pump run) (**Fig. 3**). The need for a second pump run is considered when the MR jet area is more than 1.0 cm^2 or an eccentric MR jet is observed in the authors' institution.[18]

If the site and mechanism of regurgitation cannot be evaluated accurately, the surgeon may face a problem in deciding where and how to repair the second pump run. In particular, depicting the coaptation zone of the MV in the ME LAX view is sometimes difficult owing to the acoustic shadowing caused by the annuloplasty ring implanted into the annulus. When the acceleration flow by CFD cannot be detected on the ventricular side of the repaired MV and only the regurgitant jet spreading into the left atrium can be observed, transgastric (TG) LAX and short axis views should be attempted (**Fig. 4**). The coaptation zone of the MV and subvalvular structures can often be clearly

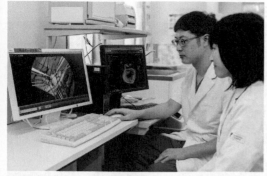

Fig. 1. Electronic medical records system that enables viewing of real-time surgical field in an echocardiographic laboratory, allowing efficient real-time information sharing between surgeons and echocardiographers.

visualized in TG views; therefore, the detection of the acceleration flow becomes easier.

Checkpoint 2: Leaflet Mobility and Alignment

It is necessary to simultaneously observe leaflet mobility and state of coaptation while searching for regurgitation using CFD. The ME LAX view and mitral commissural view by clockwise and counterclockwise probe rotation are applied for the assessment of leaflet appearance and motion. The leaflets' height should be aligned neatly next to or opposite each other with no coaptation gaps in systole. Additionally, an assessment of the degree and level of coaptation is essential; a successfully repaired MV should have a leaflet

coaptation length of 5 to 8 mm at the A2 to P2 level (**Fig. 5**).[19]

Checkpoint 3: Systolic Anterior Motion

SAM refers to the dynamic movement of the MV toward the interventricular septum during systole, resulting in left ventricular outflow tract obstruction and/or MR. Because postrepair SAM is well-known to occur in 1% to 16% of patients undergoing MV repair,[20–23] the presence of SAM immediately after repair must therefore be excluded in the ME LAX view. Excessive anterior or posterior leaflet tissues, a small and hyperkinetic left ventricle, bulging of the basal interventricular septum, and the use of a small annuloplasty ring have been identified as risk factors for SAM.[24–26] When SAM is observed during weaning from the CPB, the initial management strategy should focus on ventricular volume loading, discontinuation of inotropes, use of beta-blockers, and increasing the afterload.[27] The effects of these treatments can be observed immediately in the same ME LAX view. If significant SAM is persistent despite these medical treatments, further surgical revision is required, including reduction of the posterior leaflet's height, shortening of the neo-chords, and the use of a larger annuloplasty ring or band (**Fig. 6**).

When assessing the presence of SAM, it is important to ensure that all left ventricular segments begin to contract normally. Air embolism in the right coronary artery is a common

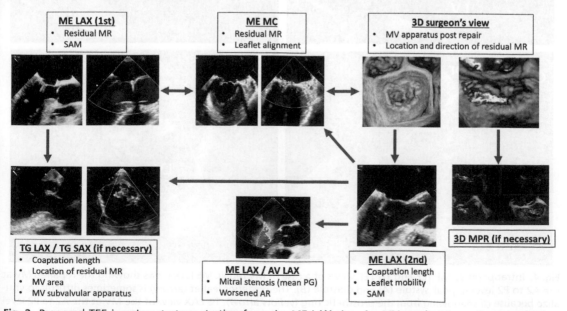

Fig. 2. Proposed TEE imaging strategy starting from the ME LAX view for MV repair. AR, aortic regurgitation; LAX, long axis; MC, mitral commissural; MPR, multiplanar reconstruction; SAX, short axis; TG, transgastric.

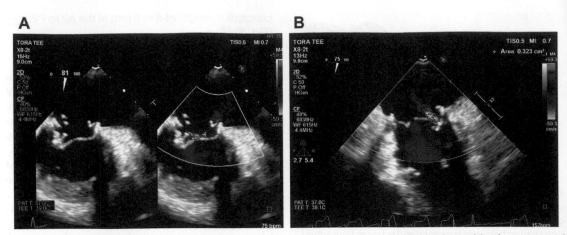

Fig. 3. Example of postrepair eccentric MR jets owing to incomplete repair. (*A*) Midesophageal (ME) commissural view showing eccentric MR toward the prosthetic ring caused by residual P3 prolapse. (*B*) ME commissural view showing eccentric MR caused by residual P1 prolapse.

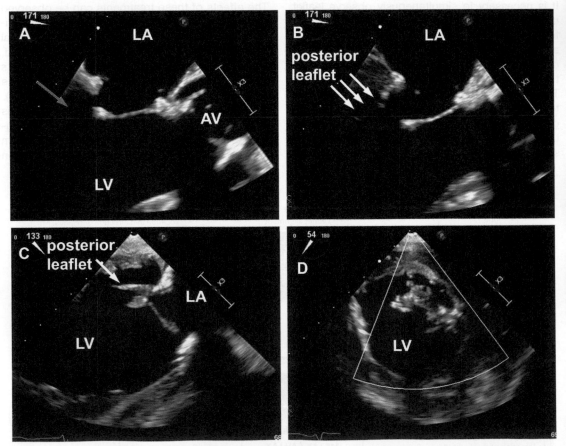

Fig. 4. Intraoperative ME TEE and TG TEE views of a case of MV repair. ME LAX views showing the repaired MV at the A2 to P2 level in peak systole (*A*) and diastole (*B*). The posterior leaflet (*arrow*) is sometimes difficult to visualize because of shadowing from the prosthetic ring (*yellow arrow*). TG LAX view of the MV at the A2 to P2 level in systole (*C*), which clearly shows the coaptation surface of the MV. The acceleration flow of residual MR can be observed with CFD in the TG short axis view of the MV at the orifice level (*D*).

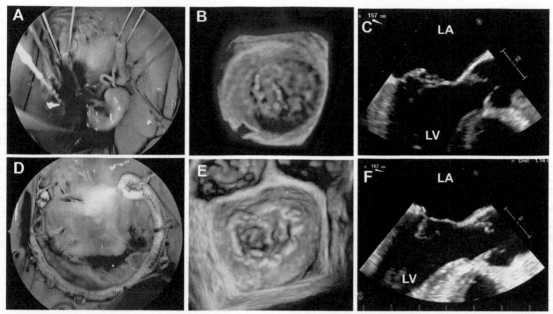

Fig. 5. A successful case of MV repair for P2 prolapse. Representative images of the MV before (*upper row; A–C*) and after (*lower row; D–F*) repair for severe MR owing to P2 prolapse. (*A*) Endoscopic view of the MV with P2 prolapse and torn chordae after placing sutures within the annulus. (*B*) A 3D photorealistic TEE surgeon's view ("TrueVue") showing a frail P2 segment and ruptured chordae tendineae. (*C*) Preoperative 2D ME LAX view showing a P2 prolapse with torn chordae. (*D*) Endoscopic view of the MV after repair during the saline test. (*E*) Intraoperative 3D TEE surgeon's view of the MV after repair at the time when the CPB was weaned off. (*F*) Postoperative 2D ME LAX view showing the coaptation surface at the A2 to P2 level.

complication immediately after CPB, which can lead to left ventricular inferior and posterior wall hypokinesis with ST-segment elevation in inferior the electrocardiographic leads (II, III, and aVF). Transient abnormalities in inferior or posterior wall motion decrease the function of papillary muscles and the mobility of the mitral posterior leaflet, thereby masking the presence of SAM. Left ventricular dyssynchrony is another component that may mask postrepair SAM. Temporary epicardial pacing is routinely used to facilitate weaning from the CPB. In several cases, TEE under pacing (often around 80–90 ppm) is forced to be continued owing to the difficulty in achieving adequate sinus rhythm and sudden atrioventricular block immediately after termination from the CPB. Nonetheless, cardiac contraction often shows a nonphysiologic pattern during ventricular

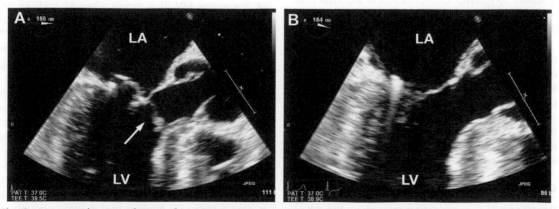

Fig. 6. An example case of SAM after MV repair requiring a second pump run and re-repair. Zoomed ME LAX views of the MV showing postrepair SAM (*arrow*) owing to excessive posterior leaflet tissue (*left, A*) and post-re-repair with shortening of the neochords after the second pump run (*right, B*).

pacing. Furthermore, there are cases in which delayed posterolateral wall contraction is generated and the posterior leaflet does not sufficiently move during systole owing to left ventricular dyssynchrony. In such cases, a significant SAM may occur as soon as an effective sinus rhythm is established. Hence, careful assessment with TEE is required because SAM may be masked when temporary cardiac pacing is indicated or the left ventricular wall motion is abnormal.

Checkpoint 4: Mitral Stenosis

The evaluation of the transvalvular flow across the MV immediately after surgery is important. Iatrogenic mitral stenosis is a recognized complication after MV repair.[28,29] Irrespective of technique, prosthetic ring or band annuloplasty is the mainstay of all repair procedures.[30] Rings or bands are used to improve the durability of repair and prevent further annular dilatation by decreasing the anatomic MV area; therefore, some degree of mitral stenosis will occur after MV repair with annuloplasty.[12,31] However, there exist no specific echocardiographic criteria for the intraoperative diagnosis of iatrogenic mitral stenosis after MV repair. Functional mitral stenosis is currently defined as an MV area of 1.5 cm^2 or less or a mean transmitral pressure gradient of 5 mm Hg or greater, irrespective of etiology. Although measurement of the anatomic MV area using 2-dimensional (2D) planimetry in the TG short axis view is useful for experienced echocardiologists, it is rarely conducted owing to technical challenges, especially in the intraoperative setting. Moreover, it is difficult to determine whether the TG short axis view is obtained at the tip level of the repaired MV and represents the smallest MV orifice area.[32] Consequently, most cardiologists and surgeons tend to rely on the mean transmitral pressure gradient to assess functional mitral stenosis after repair; nevertheless, hemodynamic changes immediately after the CPB affect this parameter.

The incidence of acute iatrogenic mitral stenosis during surgery remains unclear because the available parameters for MV area quantification in the setting immediately after repair have a different physiology, as compared with native valves. Postrepair acute mitral stenosis is rare, unless a ring that is, too small or an edge-to-edge procedure is used in multiple locations of the degenerative MV.

Checkpoint 5: Worsened Aortic Regurgitation

Postrepair TEE examination may show the emergence of a new aortic regurgitation or deterioration in preexisting aortic insufficiency if the aortic valve is injured or distorted during MV and/or tricuspid valve repair or replacement.[33–35] This iatrogenic injury to the aortic valve results from its anatomic proximity to the mitral annulus and annuloplasty ring stitches. The anterior mitral annulus is closely related to the aortic valve, specifically to the left and noncoronary aortic cusps. Normally, the distance between the nadir of these cusps and the anterior MV annulus is 5 to 10 mm; however, anatomic variations in the position of the nadir of the aortic valve and unintentional stitches may occur, resulting in suture needle perforation of the aortic cusp. Furthermore, tension caused by the MV annuloplasty ring or tricuspid valve replacement may lead to distortion of the aortic annulus owing to its adjacent position.[36] Thus, close attention should be paid to the emergence of a new aortic regurgitation after MV repair.

THE ROLE OF 3-DIMENSIONAL TRANSESOPHAGEAL ECHOCARDIOGRAPHY IN THE ASSESSMENT OF MITRAL VALVE REPAIR

Multiplane imaging with 2D TEE provides detailed assessment of cross-sectional valve anatomy and function. Although multiple thin 2D images can be mentally reconstructed into a 3D valve model, this process requires physicians to be skilled in acquiring 2D valve images with correct alignment of imaging planes according to a systematic imaging algorithm.[37] Real-time 3D TEE has improved and provided incremental value to the assessment of anatomic features, location, and extent of MV pathology.[38–41] Additionally, 3D TEE with CFD aids in identifying the location of the regurgitant orifice and direction of the regurgitant flow (**Fig. 7**). Real-time, single-beat 3D imaging is less operator dependent and enables the visualization of the entire MV in a single view as well as an assessment of the MV apparatus from either the left atrial or left ventricular perspective.[42,43] Furthermore, 3D TEE is superior to 2D TEE with respect to the identification of dominant lesions in patients with complex prolapse involving Barlow's disease and/or commissural lesions (**Fig. 8**).[44] The amount of commissural tissues varies greatly, and commissures sometimes exist as distinct leaflet scallops. In addition, 3D TEE is useful for recognizing the indentations that separate the posterior leaflet into 3 individual scallops.[45,46] The location of these indentations considerably varies among individuals, and there is also a bulky P3 scallop that is large enough to occupy the position of the original P2 segment (**Fig. 9**). This recognition is essential when planning

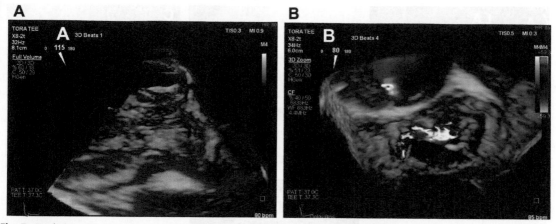

Fig. 7. Real-time 3D TG LAX view can easily shows the coaptation zone of the MV with only a single-beat acquisition (*A*). 3D multi-beat CFD of repaired MV can demonstrates an eccentric jet from P3 segment (*B*).

procedures such as indentation closure in MV repair.

Acquisition of 3D datasets is mandatory, which is ideal when assessing complex structures of the MV apparatus in detail. Multibeat, wide angle, full-volume 3D imaging can provide images with greater temporal and spatial resolution.[3,45] Nonetheless, multibeat 3D imaging requires electrocardiographic-gated acquisition and breath holds to minimize stitch artifacts, and it takes considerable experience for echocardiographers to capture high-quality 3D TEE images without artifacts.

Performing TEE for detailed preoperative evaluation in the operating room is not recommended because electrocautery-induced electrical interference has a negative effect on electrocardiographic-gated images and echocardiographic image quality is likely to be poor owing to the patients' supine position instead of left lateral position.

Surgeons have ethical duties to explain planned procedures to patients and obtain valid informed consent from patients before surgery. Therefore, preoperative TEE should be completed in the echocardiographic laboratory rather than in the operating room on the day of surgery. Furthermore, 3D TEE facilitates communication with surgeons by providing images that they may see upon opening up the left atrium in the operating

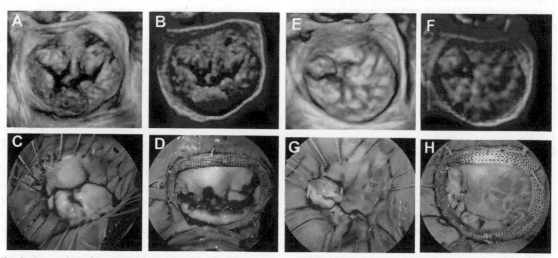

Fig. 8. Examples of Barlow's disease and commissural lesion. Representative cases of severe MR owing to Barlow's disease (*A–D*) and commissural lesion (*E–H*) are shown in 3D TEE images and endoscopic views before and after repair. Preoperative 3D surgeon's view from the left atrial perspective (*A, E*). Photorealistic 3D surgeon's view (*B, F*). Preoperative endoscopic view (*C, G*). Postoperative endoscopic view immediately after repair during the saline test (*D, H*).

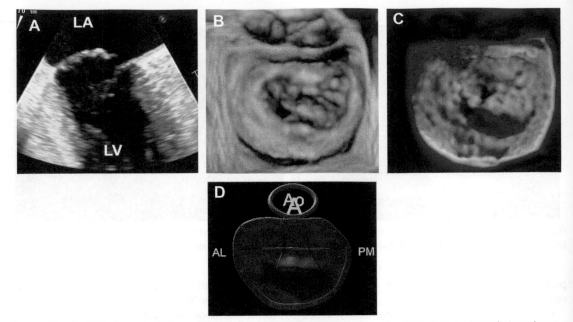

Fig. 9. A bulky P3 lesion mimicking a P2 lesion in conventional 2D images. The 2D ME commissural view shows a huge P3 lesion that is about to reach the P1 segment over the original P2 segment (*A*). These 3D surgeon's views are more intuitive for understanding the anatomic characteristics and mechanism of regurgitation (*B*). A 3D photorealistic view ("TrueVue") provides additional anatomic details (*C*). Peak systolic parametric map derived from a 3D TEE image showing prolapse of the huge P3 scallop over the P2 scallop area (*D*).

room. Further advancements in imaging will continue to improve the understanding about MV function and dysfunction both before and after repair.

SUMMARY

TEE is an important preoperative imaging modality for successful MV repair and an essential guiding tool for intraoperative decision-making among surgeons by providing immediate diagnostic feedback and assessment of results during valve repair procedures. Systematic echocardiographic evaluation of MV repair and use of 3D TEE in combination with 2D TEE based on a specific algorithm are mandatory.

CLINICS CARE POINTS

- Successful mitral valve (MV) repair is defined as a decrease in mitral regurgitation (MR) severity to mild or less without mitral stenosis (MS) or systolic anterior motion (SAM).
- Intraoperative transesophageal echocardiography (TEE) has become an essential guiding tool for decision-making among surgeons.
- Systematic echocardiographic evaluation according to the following checkpoints, including residual MR, leaflet mobility and alignment, SAM, iatrogenic MS, and worsened aortic

regurgitation should be performed immediately after MV repair.

REFERENCES

1. David TE, Armstrong S, McCrindle BW, et al. Late outcomes of mitral valve repair for mitral regurgitation due to degenerative disease. Circulation 2013; 127:1485–92.
2. Nishimura RA, Otto CM, Bonow RO, et al. Thomas JD and American College of Cardiology/American Heart Association Task Force on practice G. 2014 AHA/ACC guideline for the management of patients with valvular heart disease: executive summary: a report of the American College of Cardiology/American Heart Association Task Force on practice guidelines. J Am Coll Cardiol 2014;63: 2438–88.
3. Nicoara A, Skubas N, Ad N, et al. Guidelines for the use of transesophageal echocardiography to assist with surgical decision-making in the operating room: a surgery-based approach: from the American Society of Echocardiography in Collaboration with the Society of Cardiovascular Anesthesiologists and the Society of Thoracic Surgeons. J Am Soc Echocardiogr 2020;33:692–734.
4. La Canna G, Arendar I, Maisano F, et al. Real-time three-dimensional transesophageal echocardiography for assessment of mitral valve functional

anatomy in patients with prolapse-related regurgitation. Am J Cardiol 2011;107:1365–74.

5. Ahmed S, Nanda NC, Miller AP, et al. Usefulness of transesophageal three-dimensional echocardiography in the identification of individual segment/scallop prolapse of the mitral valve. Echocardiography 2003;20:203–9.

6. Ben Zekry S, Nagueh SF, Little SH, et al. Comparative accuracy of two- and three-dimensional transthoracic and transesophageal echocardiography in identifying mitral valve pathology in patients undergoing mitral valve repair: initial observations. J Am Soc Echocardiogr 2011;24:1079–85.

7. Mahmood F, Matyal R. A quantitative approach to the intraoperative echocardiographic assessment of the mitral valve for repair. Anesth Analg 2015;121:34–58.

8. Shah PM, Raney AA, Duran CM, et al. Multiplane transesophageal echocardiography: a roadmap for mitral valve repair. J Heart Valve Dis 1999;8:625–9.

9. Sidebotham DA, Allen SJ, Gerber IL, et al. Intraoperative transesophageal echocardiography for surgical repair of mitral regurgitation. J Am Soc Echocardiogr 2014;27:345–66.

10. Hahn RT, Abraham T, Adams MS, et al, American Society of E and Society of Cardiovascular A. Guidelines for performing a comprehensive transesophageal echocardiographic examination: recommendations from the American Society of Echocardiography and the Society of Cardiovascular Anesthesiologists. Anesth Analg 2014;118:21–68.

11. Adams DH, Anyanwu AC, Sugeng L, et al. Degenerative mitral valve regurgitation: surgical echocardiography. Curr Cardiol Rep 2008;10:226–32.

12. Ibrahim MF, David TE. Mitral stenosis after mitral valve repair for non-rheumatic mitral regurgitation. Ann Thorac Surg 2002;73:34–6.

13. Zoghbi WA, Adams D, Bonow RO, et al. Recommendations for noninvasive evaluation of native valvular regurgitation: a report from the American Society of echocardiography Developed in Collaboration with the Society for Cardiovascular Magnetic Resonance. J Am Soc Echocardiogr 2017;30:303–71.

14. Brinster DR, Unic D, D'Ambra MN, et al. Midterm results of the edge-to-edge technique for complex mitral valve repair. Ann Thorac Surg 2006;81:1612–7.

15. Riegel AK, Busch R, Segal S, et al. Evaluation of transmitral pressure gradients in the intraoperative echocardiographic diagnosis of mitral stenosis after mitral valve repair. PLoS One 2011;6:e26559.

16. Kasegawa H, Shimokawa T, Horai T, et al. Long-term echocardiography results of mitral valve repair for mitral valve prolapse. J Heart Valve Dis 2008;17:162–7.

17. Suri RM, Clavel MA, Schaff HV, et al. Effect of recurrent mitral regurgitation following degenerative mitral valve repair: long-term analysis of competing outcomes. J Am Coll Cardiol 2016;67:488–98.

18. Tabata M, Kasegawa H, Fukui T, et al. Long-term outcomes of artificial chordal replacement with tourniquet technique in mitral valve repair: a single-center experience of 700 cases. J Thorac Cardiovasc Surg 2014;148:2033–2038 e1.

19. Uchimuro T, Tabata M, Saito K, et al. Post-repair coaptation length and durability of mitral valve repair for posterior mitral valve prolapse. Gen Thorac Cardiovasc Surg 2014;62:221–7.

20. Ibrahim M, Rao C, Ashrafian H, et al. Modern management of systolic anterior motion of the mitral valve. Eur J Cardiothorac Surg 2012;41:1260–70.

21. Jebara VA, Mihaileanu S, Acar C, et al. Left ventricular outflow tract obstruction after mitral valve repair. Results of the sliding leaflet technique. Circulation 1993;88:II30–4.

22. Lee KS, Stewart WJ, Lever HM, et al. Mechanism of outflow tract obstruction causing failed mitral valve repair. Anterior displacement of leaflet coaptation. Circulation 1993;88:II24–9.

23. Crescenzi G, Landoni G, Zangrillo A, et al. Management and decision-making strategy for systolic anterior motion after mitral valve repair. J Thorac Cardiovasc Surg 2009;137:320–5.

24. Maslow AD, Regan MM, Haering JM, et al. Echocardiographic predictors of left ventricular outflow tract obstruction and systolic anterior motion of the mitral valve after mitral valve reconstruction for myxomatous valve disease. J Am Coll Cardiol 1999;34:2096–104.

25. Shah PM, Raney AA. Echocardiographic correlates of left ventricular outflow obstruction and systolic anterior motion following mitral valve repair. J Heart Valve Dis 2001;10:302–6.

26. Manabe S, Kasegawa H, Fukui T, et al. Morphological analysis of systolic anterior motion after mitral valve repair. Interact Cardiovasc Thorac Surg 2012;15:235–9.

27. Brown ML, Abel MD, Click RL, et al. Systolic anterior motion after mitral valve repair: is surgical intervention necessary? J Thorac Cardiovasc Surg 2007;133:136–43.

28. Maslow A. Mitral valve repair: an echocardiographic review: part 2. J Cardiothorac Vasc Anesth 2015;29:439–71.

29. Essandoh M. Intraoperative echocardiographic assessment of mitral valve area after degenerative mitral valve repair: a call for guidelines or recommendations. J Cardiothorac Vasc Anesth 2016;30:1364–8.

30. Bothe W, Miller DC, Doenst T. Sizing for mitral annuloplasty: where does science stop and voodoo begin? Ann Thorac Surg 2013;95:1475–83.

31. Mesana TG, Lam BK, Chan V, et al. Clinical evaluation of functional mitral stenosis after mitral valve repair for degenerative disease: potential affect on

surgical strategy. J Thorac Cardiovasc Surg 2013; 146:1418–23 [discussion: 1423–5].

32. Maslow A, Mahmood F, Poppas A, et al. Three-dimensional echocardiographic assessment of the repaired mitral valve. J Cardiothorac Vasc Anesth 2014;28:11–7.

33. Hill AC, Bansal RC, Razzouk AJ, et al. Echocardiographic recognition of iatrogenic aortic valve leaflet perforation. Ann Thorac Surg 1997;64:684–9.

34. Rother A, Smith B, Adams DH, et al. Transesophageal echocardiographic diagnosis of acute aortic valve insufficiency after mitral valve repair. Anesth Analg 2000;91:499–500.

35. Lakew F, Urbanski PP. Aortic valve leaflet perforation after minimally invasive mitral valve repair. Ann Thorac Surg 2016;101:1180–2.

36. Veronesi F, Caiani EG, Sugeng L, et al. Effect of mitral valve repair on mitral-aortic coupling: a real-time three-dimensional transesophageal echocardiography study. J Am Soc Echocardiogr 2012;25:524–31.

37. Poelaert JI, Bouchez S. Perioperative echocardiographic assessment of mitral valve regurgitation: a comprehensive review. Eur J Cardiothorac Surg 2016;50:801–12.

38. Tsang W, Weinert L, Sugeng L, et al. The value of three-dimensional echocardiography derived mitral valve parametric maps and the role of experience in the diagnosis of pathology. J Am Soc Echocardiogr 2011;24:860–7.

39. Chandra S, Salgo IS, Sugeng L, et al. Characterization of degenerative mitral valve disease using morphologic analysis of real-time three-dimensional echocardiographic images: objective insight into complexity and planning of mitral valve repair. Circ Cardiovasc Imaging 2011;4:24–32.

40. Drake DH, Zimmerman KG, Hepner AM, et al. Echo-guided mitral repair. Circ Cardiovasc Imaging 2014; 7:132–41.

41. Maffessanti F, Marsan NA, Tamborini G, et al. Quantitative analysis of mitral valve apparatus in mitral valve prolapse before and after annuloplasty: a three-dimensional intraoperative transesophageal study. J Am Soc Echocardiogr 2011;24:405–13.

42. Grewal J, Suri R, Mankad S, et al. Mitral annular dynamics in myxomatous valve disease: new insights with real-time 3-dimensional echocardiography. Circulation 2010;121:1423–31.

43. Lang RM, Badano LP, Tsang W, et al, American Society of E and European Association of E. EAE/ASE recommendations for image acquisition and display using three-dimensional echocardiography. Eur Heart J Cardiovasc Imaging 2012;13:1–46.

44. Tsang W, Lang RM. Three-dimensional echocardiography is essential for intraoperative assessment of mitral regurgitation. Circulation 2013;128:643–52 [discussion: 652].

45. Ring L, Rana BS, Ho SY, et al. The prevalence and impact of deep clefts in the mitral leaflets in mitral valve prolapse. Eur Heart J Cardiovasc Imaging 2013;14:595–602.

46. Mantovani F, Clavel MA, Vatury O, et al. Cleft-like indentations in myxomatous mitral valves by three-dimensional echocardiographic imaging. Heart 2015;101:1111–7.

Multimodality Imaging for the Assessment of Mitral Valve Disease

Dae-Hee Kim, MD, PhD

KEYWORDS

• Mitral valve • Echocardiography • Magnetic resonance imaging • Computed tomography

KEY POINTS

- The mitral valve complex's proper function needs the integrity of leaflets, annulus, chordae, papillary muscles, ventricle, and atrium. Functional, structural, or geometric distortion of one or more of these parts may cause valvular dysfunction. Therefore, comprehensive evaluations of these parameters with any imaging modality are crucial.
- Echocardiography is the primary imaging modality for visualizing the mitral valve. Three-dimensional (3D) imaging provides incremental value in assessing the severity of valvular heart disease and establishing its mechanism. For patients undergoing transcatheter intervention, real-time 3D images facilitate manipulating the catheter, to position and orient the device.
- Roles of computed tomography and cardiac MRI (CMR) are increasing. The utility of CMR for the evaluation of mitral regurgitation has recently been adopted as part of the guideline.

INTRODUCTION

The burden of valvular heart disease is increases with age. Mitral valve (MV) disease is the most common valvular heart disease. The prevalence in subjects older than 75 years is almost 10%.[1] Imaging is needed to assess or be evaluated for (1) valve morphology to determine the etiology (anatomic assessment), (2) valve function and the severity of valvular heart disease (hemodynamic assessment), (3) remodeling of the left ventricle (LV) and right ventricle (RV), and (4) preplanning and guidance of percutaneous intervention. Echocardiography is the primary imaging modality for visualizing the MV. Although roles of computed tomography (CT) and cardiac magnetic resonance (CMR) are increasing, echocardiography serves as the first-line imaging modality for diagnosis and serial follow-up in most cases. This review summarizes the roles of multimodality imaging currently available from research fields to daily clinical practice.

NORMAL MITRAL VALVE ANATOMY

The MV apparatus comprises an annulus, 2 leaflets, chordae tendineae, and papillary muscles (**Fig. 1**).[2] The MV annulus, a D-shaped ring rather than circular shape positioned in the left atrioventricular groove, extends from 2 fibrous trigones located at either end of the area of fibrous continuity between the aortic leaflet of the MV and the aortic root.[3] This straight border forms the anterior part of the annulus, which is in fibrous continuity with the aortic valve. The remaining border of the annulus forms the posterior annulus. Annular remodeling occurs predominantly in the posterior part of the annulus (asymmetric annular dilation), because the posterior part of the annulus faces pliant endocardium, not a fibrous skeleton.[4]

Anterior and posterior mitral leaflets are not equal in size.[5] The anterior leaflet attaches to one-third of the annulus but encloses a larger portion of the valve orifice than the posterior leaflet dose. The anterior leaflet is one of the parts of LV outflow tract

Division of Cardiology, Asan Medical Center, College of Medicine, University of Ulsan, 388-1, Poongnap-dong, Songpa-ku, Seoul 138-736, Korea
E-mail address: daehee74@amc.seoul.kr

Cardiol Clin 39 (2021) 243–253
https://doi.org/10.1016/j.ccl.2021.01.007
0733-8651/21/© 2021 Elsevier Inc. All rights reserved.

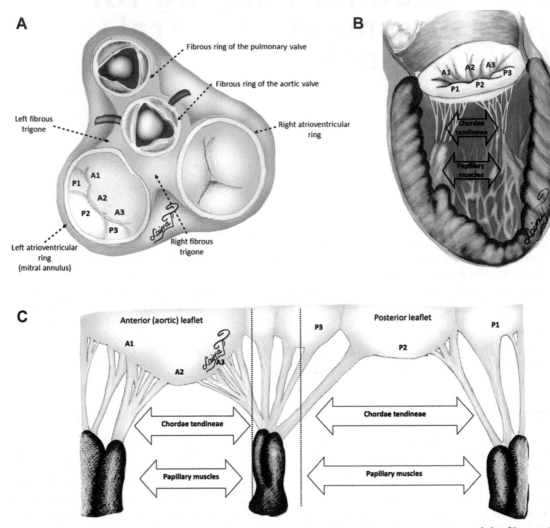

Fig. 1. Anatomy of the MV apparatus. Craniocaudal view of the heart (*A*) with components of the fibrous skeleton. Longitudinal cross-sectional view (*B*) highlighting the position of the MV, chordae tendineae and PMs. Expanded view of the MV leaflets, chordae, and proximal parts of the PMs (*C*). (*From* Tumenas A, Tamkeviciute L, Arzanauskiene R, Arzanauskaite M. Multimodality Imaging of the Mitral Valve: Morphology, Function, and Disease. *Current Problems in Diagnostic Radiology.* 2020; with permission.)

(LVOT) during systole, causing outflow tract obstruction in hypertrophic obstructive cardiomyopathy.[6] Three segments form each leaflet: A1, A2, and A3 in the anterior leaflet and P1, P2, and P3 in the posterior leaflet. The clefts or indentations along the free margin of the posterior leaflet make it a scalloped appearance. Despite the absence of indentations, similar terminology is applied for the anterior leaflet scallops. Three scallops are not equal in size, and middle scallops are larger in most cases.[7] When the leaflets coapt during diastole, the view of the valve from the atrium resembles a smile. Each end of the coaptation line is named as a commissure. Normally, the valvar leaflets are thin, translucent, and soft, and each leaflet has an atrial and a ventricular surface.

The MV leaflets are braced by chordae, and attach to 2 papillary muscles (PMs). The tendinous cords are stringlike structures that connect the ventricular surface or the free edge of the leaflets to the PMs.[8] The first-order cords are inserted into the free edge of the MV. Second-order cords insert on the ventricular surface of the leaflets beyond the free edge, forming the rough zone. Third-order cords are connected only to the mural leaflet because they arise directly from the ventricular wall.[8] The Toronto group classified them into leaflets and interleaflet or commissural cords.[9] Viewed from the atrial aspect, the 2 PMs are located below the commissures, positioning in anterolateral and posteromedial directions. The anterolateral PM is a single in 70% of cases, and the posteromedial PM is 2 or 3 in number or 1 PM with 2 or 3 heads in 60%.[8]

Echocardiography

Transthoracic echocardiography (TTE) is the first-line imaging modality for screening, assessment, diagnosis, and surveillance of valvular disease. For MV disease, TTE is still the mainstream for evaluating the etiology, anatomic morphology, and grade of mitral regurgitation (MR) or stenosis (MS). The proper function of the MV complex needs the integrity of leaflets, mitral annulus, chordae, PMs, LV, and left atrium (LA). Functional, structural, or geometric distortion of 1 or more of these parts may cause valvular dysfunction.[10] The grading of severity of valvular heart disease will not be discussed herein. Comprehensive approaches with multimodality imaging are especially required for the assessment of MR.[11]

Three-dimensional (3D) imaging provides incremental value in the assessment of severity of valvular stenosis (**Fig. 2**A) or regurgitation (**Fig. 2**B) and in establishing its mechanism. Traditionally, two-dimensional (2D) imaging requires multiple view acquisitions, including modified views of the MV, to make a detailed assessment of MV morphology, adjuring longer study time and expert interpretation. Three-dimensional

transesophageal echocardiography (TEE) has become widely used in operating rooms and cardiac catheterization laboratories. Three-dimensional TEE has been proven to be superior to 2D TEE in the assessment of both MV anatomy and MR.[12] One reason for this superiority is that 3D TEE allows the MV to be visualized en face in an orientation identical to the surgeon's view of the MV intraoperatively (**Fig. 2**B, C), and 3D TEE enables the person with relatively little training to acquire high-quality real-time 3D images even in a single beat. Three-dimensional echocardiography has multiple acquisition modes and display options (simultaneous multiplane imaging, tomographic slices, surface rendering, and volume rendering); moreover, simultaneous 2D multiplane imaging ("x-plane or biplane mode") in a modifiable angulation.[13] Accurate preoperative or preprocedural assessment of the valve anatomy and location of lesions are critical in the management of patients with severe MR.[14] This information determines whether the patient should undergo valve repair or replacement and influences the timing of surgery accordingly.

For patients undergoing transcatheter intervention for MR, adequate patient selection for these therapies requires a precise assessment of MV anatomy and function. Moreover, live 3D TEE en face views of the MV facilitate manipulation of

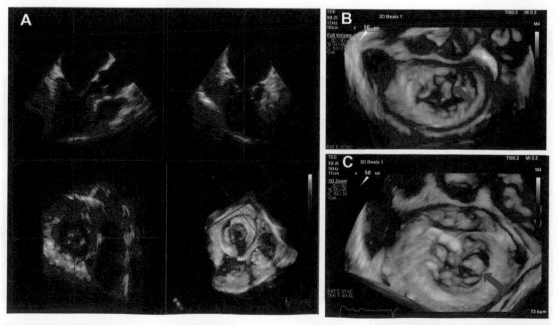

Fig. 2. Multiplanar reconstruction (MPR) mode on 3D TEE to assess the MV. Using MPR mode in patients with mitral stenosis allows a more accurate valve measurement (*A*). Three-dimensional reconstruction of the MV en face in an orientation identical to the surgeon's view shows A2 prolapse with ruptured chordae (*red arrow, B*). Three-dimensional en face view depicting a medical commissural prolapse (*red arrow, C*). Differentiation between commissural prolapse and A3, P3 prolapse is crucial in the era of the MV intervention.

the catheter, to position and orient the device without damaging adjacent structures (**Fig. 3**A, B). The biplane (x-plane) views show simultaneously the bi-commissural, and the 3-chamber long-axis planes (**Fig. 3**C) is most frequently used to fine-tune the orientation of the device relative to the largest regurgitant orifice area and perpendicular to the coaptation line.

Further anatomic or geometric qualifications with echocardiography

In patients with hypertrophic cardiomyopathy, LV outflow tract obstruction (LVOTO) is produced by systolic anterior motion of the MV. Clinical implications of MV size in hypertrophic cardiomyopathy have been elucidated with 2D and 3D echocardiography, which recently allowed mitral leaflet size and area in the beating heart (**Fig. 4**).[15,16] In vivo measurement of mitral leaflet area makes it possible to understand more on the mechanisms of ischemic/function MR in detail using 3D echocardiography.[4,17,18] Recently, commercialized software supports the measurement.[19,20]

The visualization of mitral annulus shape using 3D echocardiography has contributed to the development of nonplanar mitral annuloplasty rings.[21] Comprehensive analysis of annulus geometry, including area, perimeter, nonplanar angle, diameters, intertrigone distance, and height can provide valuable information to reveal the mechanism of valvular heart disease (**Fig. 5**).[22,23] Minimal mitral annulus dimensions are present in early systole, and annulus dimensions increase toward late systole. Changes in all parameters acquired from annulus geometry can be calculated during the cardiac cycle; annular dynamics differ between healthy subjects and patients with MV disease.[24]

Computed Tomography Scan

Cardiac CT scan acquires the images with the injection of contrast agents, and protocol is structured to allow assessment of the coronary arteries as well. The pathologic imaging findings of the MV including prolapse, vegetation, and coaptation gap, can be well demonstrated in the systolic phase of the cardiac cycle. Cine reconstruction methods using volume-rendered images are useful for visualizing MV structure. At our institution, cardiac CT for evaluation of both the coronary artery and MV is performed with a second-generation dual-source CT scanner (Definition Flash; Siemens, Erlangen, Germany). The images acquired in the mid-systolic phase are used to evaluate the MV. Images are reconstructed with the 5% R-R interval (20 images per 1 cardiac cycle) for retrospective electrocardiogram (ECG)-gated scanning and at 10-ms intervals for prospective ECG-triggered scanning.[25]

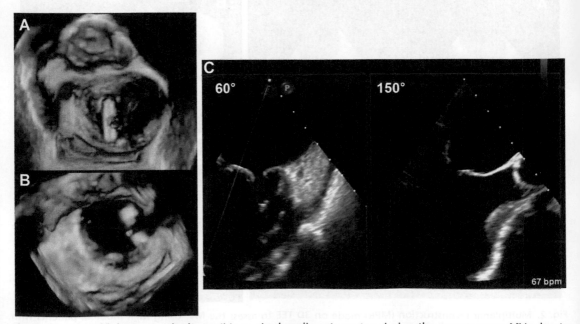

Fig. 3. Real-time 3D images make it possible to check a clip orientation during the percutaneous MV edge to edge repair (A, B). The clip is recommended to be placed perpendicular to the coaptation line. Reducing 3D gain can visualize the clip in the LV (B). X-plane imaging is advantageous to guide the percutaneous mitral intervention. The bi-commissural (*left*) and LVOT view (*right*) images are crucial for the MitraClip intervention (C).

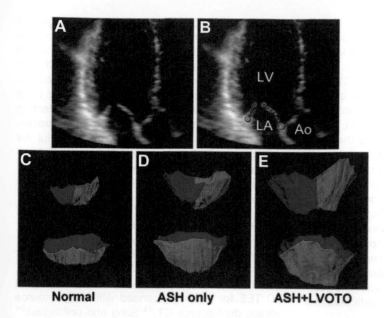

Normal **ASH only** **ASH+LVOTO**

Fig. 4. Component view with mitral leaflet traces for 3D reconstruction (*A, B*). Representative open mitral leaflet area measurements in green and purple for anterior and posterior leaflets viewed from the side (*C* through *E*, top row, lateral commissure in foreground) and LVOT aspect below, largest in asymmetric septal hypertrophy (ASH) and ASH with LVOTO. Ao, aorta. (*From* Kim DH, Handschumacher MD, Levine RA, et al. In vivo measurement of mitral leaflet surface area and subvalvular geometry in patients with asymmetrical septal hypertrophy: insights into the mechanism of outflow tract obstruction. Circulation. 2010;122(13):1298-1307; with permission.)

Assessment of prolapse segment with computed tomography scan

In our clinical practice, we review the quality of images with 4-dimensional multiphase CT data including the 3-chamber view. We found that the best-quality images were obtained during the 25% to 35% cardiac phases in approximately 80% of patients with MV prolapse.[25] A step-by-step method for the image reconstruction of MV can be summarized as follows: (1) determine the best cardiac phase; (2) identify the location and extent of disease on sagittal and coronal views of the MV by using a multiplanar reformatted technique (anterior vs posterior leaflet in the sagittal view; medial, middle, or lateral scallops in the coronal view); and (3) recheck the extent and location

of the disease on the 3D volume-rendered image (**Fig. 6**).[25]

The localization of the MV prolapse segment is feasible on a per-scallop basis, but it may underestimate the extent of prolapsed scallop compared with TEE, particularly in patients with multiple-scallop lesions. The per-scallop sensitivity of cardiac CT was slightly lower than that of echocardiography (80% vs 87%, $P = .004$), with similar specificity (both 95%).[26]

Detection of paravalvular leakage in patients with prosthetic heart valve

Paravalvular leakage (PVL) is defined as an abnormal communication between the sewing ring and valve annulus and the prevalence of

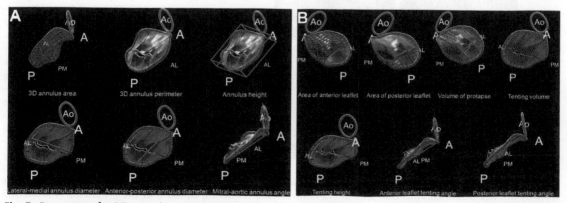

Fig. 5. Parameters for MV annulus geometry (*A*). Parameters for MV leaflet geometry (*B*). A, anterior; AL, anterolateral; Ao, aortic annulus; P, posterior; PM, posteromedial. (*From* Song JM, Jung YJ, Jung YJ, et al. Three-dimensional remodeling of mitral valve in patients with significant regurgitation secondary to rheumatic versus prolapse etiology. Am J Cardiol. 2013;111(11):1631-1637; with permission.)

PVL after MV replacement ranges from 3% to 15%.[27] For severe symptomatic PVL, surgical corrections perform either repair of the leak or re-replacement have been recommended. However, the recurrence rates range from 12% to 35%, and therefore percutaneous device closure has been introduced as an alternative option to treat PVL.[28] For decision making in PVL treatment, anatomic information, including the size, shape, and the 3D relationship with adjacent structures should be considered as parts of pre-procedural planning. Echocardiography is the primary modality of choice that provides excellent temporal resolution and real-time imaging capabilities with color Doppler information, but sometimes image quality can be compromised. In contrast, cardiac CT can give more precise anatomic details, including the exact location and morphology of the PVLs. Pretreatment planning could be better tailored and individualized with cardiac CT scan (**Fig. 7**).[29]

Detection and diagnosis of infective endocarditis

Echocardiography is the imaging method of choice for the diagnosis of infective endocarditis (IE), but the operator dependency and poor sonic window caused by calcifications or detection on vegetation on mechanical prosthetic valves are still limitations. A recent meta-analysis showed that CT might provide incremental value to TEE for diagnosing prosthetic valve IE.[30] Kim and colleagues[31] reported the overall detection rate of vegetation was inferior in CT compared with TEE (97.3% vs 72.0%), but cardiac CT shows comparable diagnostic performance with TEE for large vegetation (≥10 mm). TEE was better for detecting small vegetation, valve perforation, and intracardiac fistula, whereas CT was more useful for detecting perivalvular abscess and coronary artery disease.[31] In contrast, another report showed similar sensitivities between CT and TEE to detect IE, and excellent interobserver agreement.[32]

Leaflet size, annulus geometry, and relationship with papillary muscles

Mitral leaflet area and annulus area measured by CT were comparable with 3D echocardiography, and there was no difference in agreement with 3D TEE for patients scanned with single-source versus dual-source CT.[33] Song and colleagues[34] explored geometric predictors of LVOTO in patients with hypertrophic cardiomyopathy by using cardiac CT and found that anterior mitral leaflet length and the distance between lateral PM base and LV apex were independent predictors of LVOTO. Cardiac CT has an advantage of more accurate evaluation of the 3D geometry of myocardial hypertrophy pattern and PMs than CMR and echocardiography.[29,32,34]

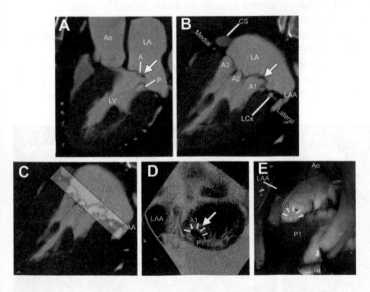

Fig. 6. Reconstruction of CT images of the MV to evaluate the extent and location of MV prolapse. A1, A2, and A3 = lateral, middle, and medial scallops of the anterior leaflet, respectively; P1, P2, and P3 = lateral, middle, and medial scallops of the posterior leaflet, respectively. Parasagittal reconstructed CT image shows MV prolapse in the A1 portion (*A*). A coronal reconstructed CT image shows a prolapsed scallop of the MV (*arrow*) near the left atrial appendage, which is a landmark of a lateral direction in the MV annulus. The proximal left circumflex artery (LCX) is also located in the lateral direction, and the coronary sinus (CS) and interatrial septum are located in the medial direction (*B*). Coronal thin-section maximum intensity projection reconstructed CT image obtained at the level of the valve shows the section thickness used to generate the surgeon's view (*C*). Surgeon's view of the MV obtained with thin-section (15-mm) volume rendering shows that the A1 scallop is prolapsed (*D*). Intraoperative photograph obtained with a robot-assisted surgery system shows that the locations of the prolapsed scallop and left atrial appendage (LAA) correspond with the CT findings (*E*). Ao, ascending aorta. (*From* Koo HJ, Yang DH, Oh SY, et al. Demonstration of mitral valve prolapse with CT for planning of mitral valve repair. Radiographics. 2014;34(6):1537-1552; with permission.)

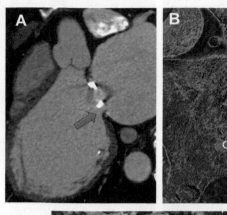

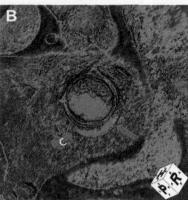

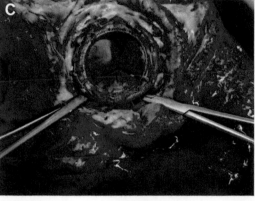

Fig. 7. Large crescent-shaped dehiscence (*yellow arrows*) that involved posterior part of the mitral annulus on CT images (*A, B*). A single large PVL in surgical inspection was confirmed. Surgical instruments indicate the medial and lateral ends of the paravalvular dehiscence (*C*).

In the ear of transcatheter MV replacement (TMVR), CT is becoming a critical imaging modality for identifying the MV anatomy and its spatial relationships with other structures. The parameters measuring the MV annulus geometry are essential to select the size of transcatheter MV annuloplasty devices and TMVR. The assessment of MV annulus calcification is essential to check the feasibility of various transcatheter therapies.[10] For TMVR planning, truncation of the saddle-shaped annular contour at a virtual line connecting both trigones (trigone-to-trigone [TT] distance), has been used.[24] Three-dimensional segmentation and post-processing yield annular area and perimeter, TT distance, septal-to-lateral distance (A2-to-P2 distance, minor diameter), and the inter-commissural (IC) distance (major diameter).[24] Similar post-processing using 3D echocardiography full-volume set can be performed off-line (**Fig. 8**).

CARDIAC MAGNETIC RESONANCE IMAGING

CMR provides a comprehensive evaluation of cardiac anatomy, function, and myocardial tissue characterization, and the usefulness to assess valvular heart disease, especially regurgitation, is increasingly recognized. The utility of CMR for the evaluation of valvular regurgitation has recently been adopted as part of the joint American Society of Echocardiography and the Society of Cardiovascular Magnetic Resonance recommendations for the noninvasive evaluation of native valvular regurgitation.[11] For assessment of the severity of MR, CMR has become an established noninvasive imaging modality to assess the severity of MR (**Fig. 9**).[35]

Valve Structure and Ventricular Function Assessment

To visualize the morphology and motion of the MV from any desired image orientation, balanced steady-state free precession (SSFP) sequence cine imaging techniques have been widely used for the evaluation of valvular structures in motion, because it can provide a high signal-to-noise ratio (excellent contrast) between the blood pool and myocardium. Older sequences such as "black blood" turbo-spin-echo (TSE) techniques (T1-weighted and T2-weighted TSE imaging techniques) can be used for the evaluation of valvular masses such as vegetations or tumors..[36]

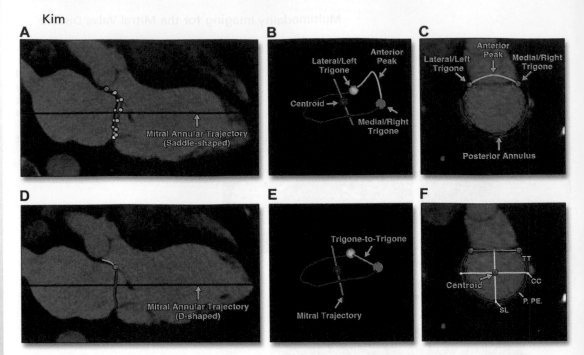

Fig. 8. Saddle-shaped annulus segmentation as a cubic spline interpolation (*A*). Pink line = anterior peak; red line = posterior peak (posterior mitral leaflet insertion, P. PE.); green and blue dots = fibrous trigones (*B*). Importantly, the anterior peak projects into the LVOT (short-axis view [*C*] and long-axis view [*D*]). The more planar D-shaped annular contour is created by truncating the saddle-shaped contour at the TT distance (*yellow lines* [*E*, *F*]). Important measurements are the projected area setal-to-lateral (SL) and intercommissural (CC) distances; the latter is oriented perpendicularly to SL while transecting through the centroid (*F*). (*From* Blanke P, Naoum C, Webb J, et al. Multimodality Imaging in the Context of Transcatheter Mitral Valve Replacement: Establishing Consensus Among Modalities and Disciplines. JACC Cardiovasc Imaging. 2015;8(10):1191-1208; with permission.)

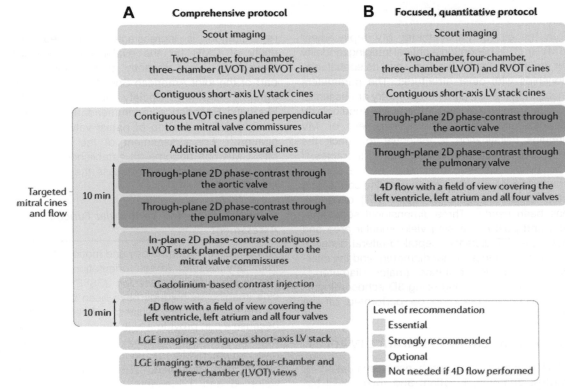

Fig. 9. Recommended cardiovascular MRI protocols for the assessment of MR. Comprehensive cardiovascular MRI protocol for the assessment of MR (*A*). Focused, quantitative protocol (*B*). LGE, late gadolinium enhancement; RVOT, right ventricular outflow tract. (*From* Garg P, Swift AJ, Zhong L, et al. Assessment of mitral valve regurgitation by cardiovascular magnetic resonance imaging. Nat Rev Cardiol. 2020;17(5):298-312; with permission.)

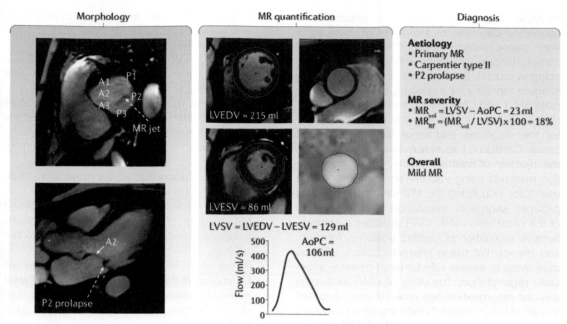

Fig. 10. MR assessment in a patient with ischemic cardiomyopathy. Incomplete coaptation owing to ventricular dilatation is seen on the short-axis cines (morphology panel, *top images*). A through-plane phase-contrast acquisition shows the central MR jet (morphology panel, *right-hand middle image*). LGE imaging reveals extensive ischemic myocardial scaring (morphology panel, *right-hand bottom image*). The MR volume (MRvol) is quantified using the standard method: LV stroke volume (LVSV) minus aortic phase-contrast forward volume (AoPC). LVEDV, left ventricular end-diastolic volume; LVESV, left ventricular end-systolic volume; MRRF, mitral regurgitation fraction. (*From* Garg P, Swift AJ, Zhong L, et al. Assessment of mitral valve regurgitation by cardiovascular magnetic resonance imaging. Nat Rev Cardiol. 2020;17(5):298-312; with permission.)

Quantification of LV size and volumes by SSFP technique of CMR can be an integral part of a comprehensive assessment as a reference method and are needed for the decision making of a treatment plan (timing of surgery). Ventricular volumes are determined from a short-axis stack of 6-mm-thick to 8-mm-thick slices. They can be analyzed with off-line software, allowing endocardial and epicardial border tracing of both ventricles automatically or manually. Likewise, the Simpson method can be used to calculate ventricular volumes, ejection fractions, and myocardial mass.[36]

Flow Visualization and Quantification

Phase-contrast velocity encoding is a technique that uses velocity-encoding (VENC) gradients to generate a phase shift in the MRI signal, which is proportional to the velocity of the moving protons.[36] Four-dimensional-flow CMR allows for visualization of 2D velocity vectors in a designated plane, enabling a comprehensive assessment of the blood flow dynamics in the LA. Velocity vector visualization of LA flow coupled with cine CMR can help to understand the cause of the MR, similar to Doppler imaging acquired

from echocardiography.[36] The MR jet cane be visualized using both cine and 2D phase-contrast CMR. Quantification of mitral regurgitant volume and fraction is the recommended technique, and the MR volume can be calculated by 4 different methods: (1) Standard method and widely used: the difference between the LV stroke volume calculated using planimetry of cine SSFP images and the aortic forward volume obtained by phase-contrast images (**Fig. 10**); (2) the difference between the LV and RV stroke volumes calculated using planimetry of cine SSFP images; (3) the difference between the mitral inflow stroke volume and the aortic forward volume; and (4) direct quantification of MR flow by 4D-flow CMR with retrospective MV tracking.[35]

For the evaluation of patients with MR, late gadolinium enhancement (LGE) imaging to test viability should be performed in accordance with published guidelines.[37] Contiguous, short-axis, LV stack LGE imaging is needed, in addition to LGE in the 3 standard long-axis planes.

SUMMARY

The MV complex's proper function needs the integrity of leaflets, annulus, chordae, PMs, ventricle, and atrium. Functional, structural, or geometric distortion of 1 or more of these parts may cause valvular dysfunction. Therefore, a comprehensive evaluation with multimodality imaging is crucial. Echocardiography is the primary imaging modality for assessing the MV. Although roles of CT and CMR are increasing, echocardiography will serve as the first-line imaging modality for the diagnosis and serial follow-up in most cases. Cardiac CT scan acquires the images with the injection of contrast agents. Cine reconstruction methods using volume-rendered images are useful for visualizing the MV structure, including prolapse segments, vegetation, and dehiscence of the prosthetic valve. CMR provides a comprehensive evaluation of cardiac anatomy, function, and myocardial tissue characterization, and the usefulness to assess valvular heart disease, especially regurgitation. The utility of CMR evaluating valvular regurgitation has recently been adopted as part of the guideline. Finally, improved accuracy in the noninvasive assessment of MV and its related structures with multimodality imaging will ultimately translate to better management to improve outcomes for patients with MV disease.

CLINICS CARE POINTS

- Echocardiography is the primary imaging modality for visualizing the mitral valve. 3D imaging provides incremental value in assessing the severity of valvular heart disease and establishing its mechanism and is crucial for the guidance of percutaneous interventions.

- Roles of computed tomography and magnetic resonance imaging (CMR) are increasing. For the assessment of mitral regurgitation severity, CMR has recently been adopted as part of the guideline and become an established noninvasive imaging modality.

DISCLOSURE

The author has nothing to disclose.

REFERENCES

1. Nkomo VT, Gardin JM, Skelton TN, et al. Burden of valvular heart diseases: a population-based study. Lancet 2006;368(9540):1005–11.
2. Tumenas A, Tamkeviciute L, Arzanauskiene R, et al. Multimodality Imaging of the Mitral Valve: Morphology, Function, and Disease. Current Problems in Diagnostic Radiology. 2020. https://doi.org/10.1067/j.cpradiol.2020.09.013.
3. Berdajs D, Zund G, Camenisch C, et al. Annulus fibrosus of the mitral valve: reality or myth. J Card Surg 2007;22(5):406–9.
4. Kim DH, Heo R, Handschumacher MD, et al. Mitral valve adaptation to isolated annular dilation: insights into the mechanism of atrial functional mitral regurgitation. JACC Cardiovasc Imaging 2019;12(4):665–77.
5. Barlow JB. Perspectives on the mitral valve. Philadelphia: F.A. Davis; 1987.
6. Morris MF, Maleszewski JJ, Suri RM, et al. CT and MR imaging of the mitral valve: radiologic-pathologic correlation. Radiographics 2010;30(6):1603–20.
7. Ranganathan N, Lam JH, Wigle ED, et al. Morphology of the human mitral valve. II. The value leaflets. Circulation 1970;41(3):459–67.
8. Ho SY. Anatomy of the mitral valve. Heart 2002;88(Suppl 4):iv5–10.
9. Lam JH, Ranganathan N, Wigle ED, et al. Morphology of the human mitral valve. I. Chordae tendineae: a new classification. Circulation 1970;41(3):449–58.
10. Bax JJ, Debonnaire P, Lancellotti P, et al. Transcatheter interventions for mitral regurgitation: multimodality imaging for patient selection and procedural guidance. JACC Cardiovasc Imaging 2019;12(10):2029–48.
11. Zoghbi WA, Adams D, Bonow RO, et al. Recommendations for noninvasive evaluation of native valvular regurgitation: a report from the American Society of Echocardiography developed in collaboration with the Society for Cardiovascular Magnetic Resonance. J Am Soc Echocardiogr 2017;30(4):303–71.
12. Tsang W, Lang RM. Three-dimensional echocardiography is essential for intraoperative assessment of mitral regurgitation. Circulation 2013;128(6):643–52 [discussion: 652].
13. Lang RM, Badano LP, Tsang W, et al. EAE/ASE recommendations for image acquisition and display using three-dimensional echocardiography. Eur Heart J Cardiovasc Imaging 2012;13(1):1–46.
14. La Canna G, Arendar I, Maisano F, et al. Real-time three-dimensional transesophageal echocardiography for assessment of mitral valve functional anatomy in patients with prolapse-related regurgitation. Am J Cardiol 2011;107(9):1365–74.
15. Klues HG, Proschan MA, Dollar AL, et al. Echocardiographic assessment of mitral valve size in obstructive hypertrophic cardiomyopathy. Anatomic validation from mitral valve specimen. Circulation 1993;88(2):548–55.
16. Kim DH, Handschumacher MD, Levine RA, et al. In vivo measurement of mitral leaflet surface area

and subvalvular geometry in patients with asymmetrical septal hypertrophy: insights into the mechanism of outflow tract obstruction. Circulation 2010; 122(13):1298–307.

17. Chaput M, Handschumacher MD, Tournoux F, et al. Mitral leaflet adaptation to ventricular remodeling: occurrence and adequacy in patients with functional mitral regurgitation. Circulation 2008;118(8): 845–52.

18. Dal-Bianco JP, Aikawa E, Bischoff J, et al. Active adaptation of the tethered mitral valve: insights into a compensatory mechanism for functional mitral regurgitation. Circulation 2009;120(4):334–42.

19. Cobey FC, Swaminathan M, Phillips-Bute B, et al. Quantitative assessment of mitral valve coaptation using three-dimensional transesophageal echocardiography. Ann Thorac Surg 2014;97(6):1998–2004.

20. Machino-Ohtsuka T, Seo Y, Ishizu T, et al. Novel mechanistic insights into atrial functional mitral regurgitation-3-dimensional echocardiographic study. Circ J 2016;80(10):2240–8.

21. Carpentier AF, Lessana A, Relland JY, et al. The "physio-ring": an advanced concept in mitral valve annuloplasty. Ann Thorac Surg 1995;60(5):1177–85 [discussion: 1185–6].

22. Lee AP, Hsiung MC, Salgo IS, et al. Quantitative analysis of mitral valve morphology in mitral valve prolapse with real-time 3-dimensional echocardiography: importance of annular saddle shape in the pathogenesis of mitral regurgitation. Circulation 2013;127(7):832–41.

23. Song JM, Jung YJ, Jung YJ, et al. Three-dimensional remodeling of mitral valve in patients with significant regurgitation secondary to rheumatic versus prolapse etiology. Am J Cardiol 2013;111(11):1631–7.

24. Blanke P, Naoum C, Webb J, et al. Multimodality imaging in the context of transcatheter mitral valve replacement: establishing consensus among modalities and disciplines. JACC Cardiovasc Imaging 2015;8(10):1191–208.

25. Koo HJ, Yang DH, Oh SY, et al. Demonstration of mitral valve prolapse with CT for planning of mitral valve repair. Radiographics 2014;34(6):1537–52.

26. Koo HJ, Kang JW, Oh SY, et al. Cardiac computed tomography for the localization of mitral valve prolapse: scallop-by-scallop comparisons with echocardiography and intraoperative findings. Eur Heart J Cardiovasc Imaging 2019;20(5):550–7.

27. Ionescu A, Fraser AG, Butchart EG. Prevalence and clinical significance of incidental paraprosthetic valvar regurgitation: a prospective study using transoesophageal echocardiography. Heart 2003; 89(11):1316–21.

28. Ruiz CE, Jelnin V, Kronzon I, et al. Clinical outcomes in patients undergoing percutaneous closure of periprosthetic paravalvular leaks. J Am Coll Cardiol 2011;58(21):2210–7.

29. Koo HJ, Lee JY, Kim GH, et al. Paravalvular leakage in patients with prosthetic heart valves: cardiac computed tomography findings and clinical features. Eur Heart J Cardiovasc Imaging 2018; 19(12):1419–27.

30. Habets J, Tanis W, Reitsma JB, et al. Are novel noninvasive imaging techniques needed in patients with suspected prosthetic heart valve endocarditis? A systematic review and meta-analysis. Eur Radiol 2015;25(7):2125–33.

31. Kim IC, Chang S, Hong GR, et al. Comparison of cardiac computed tomography with transesophageal echocardiography for identifying vegetation and intracardiac complications in patients with infective endocarditis in the era of 3-dimensional images. Circ Cardiovasc Imaging 2018;11(3): e006986.

32. Koo HJ, Yang DH, Kang JW, et al. Demonstration of infective endocarditis by cardiac CT and transesophageal echocardiography: comparison with intraoperative findings. Eur Heart J Cardiovasc Imaging 2018;19(2):199–207.

33. Beaudoin J, Thai WE, Wai B, et al. Assessment of mitral valve adaptation with gated cardiac computed tomography: validation with three-dimensional echocardiography and mechanistic insight to functional mitral regurgitation. Circ Cardiovasc Imaging 2013;6(5):784–9.

34. Song Y, Yang DH, Hartaigh BÓ, et al. Geometric predictors of left ventricular outflow tract obstruction in patients with hypertrophic cardiomyopathy: a 3D computed tomography analysis. Eur Heart J Cardiovasc Imaging 2018;19(10):1149–56.

35. Garg P, Swift AJ, Zhong L, et al. Assessment of mitral valve regurgitation by cardiovascular magnetic resonance imaging. Nat Rev Cardiol 2020; 17(5):298–312.

36. Mathew RC, Loffler AI, Salerno M. Role of cardiac magnetic resonance imaging in valvular heart disease: diagnosis, assessment, and management. Curr Cardiol Rep 2018;20(11):119.

37. Kramer CM, Barkhausen J, Bucciarelli-Ducci C, et al. Standardized cardiovascular magnetic resonance imaging (CMR) protocols: 2020 update. J Cardiovasc Magn Reson 2020;22(1):17.

Revisiting the Role of Guideline-Directed Medical Therapy for Patients with Heart Failure and Severe Functional Mitral Regurgitation

Shun Kohsaka, MD[a],*, Mike Saji, MD, PhD[b], Satoshi Shoji, MD, PhD[a],
Keisuke Matsuo, MD[c], Shintaro Nakano, MD, PhD[c],
Yuji Nagatomo, MD, PhD[d], Takashi Kohno, MD, PhD[e]

KEYWORDS

- Heart failure • Medical therapy • Mitral regurgitation • MitraClip

KEY POINTS

- Patients with heart failure often have mitral regurgitation, which can create a vicious cycle.
- Medical therapy remains the mainstay of treatment in this setting.
- This review revisits the role of medical therapy and its optimization for severe functional mitral regurgitation.

INTRODUCTION

Heart failure (HF) is a growing epidemic that affects more than 6 million adults in the United States.[1] Functional mitral regurgitation (FMR) is common in patients with HF, and reported to be prevalent in more than 16,000 cases per 1 million population.[2] FMR frequently generates a vicious cycle of worsening HF and MR, in which a dilated left ventricle from volume overload results in a dilated mitral annulus with tethered mitral leaflets (worsening of FMR), which in turn can lead to progression in HF. A recent meta-analysis of 53 studies and 45,900 patients revealed that FMR was associated with increased risks of cardiac mortality, HF hospitalization, transplantation, and death.[3]

Worsening HF and MR can be modified in several ways in the contemporary era. The valid medical interventions include medical therapy, surgical intervention, or transcatheter intervention. Medical therapy remains the mainstay of

Conflicts of Interest: S. Kohsaka received lecture fees and research grants from Bristol Myers Squibb, Bayer Yakuhin and Daiichi Sankyo. All other authors have no relevant conflict of interest to disclose.
Funding: This work was supported by the Grants-in-Aid for Scientific Research from the Japan Society for the Promotion of Science (KAKENHI; No. 25460630, 25460777, 16H05215, https://kaken.nii.ac.jp/ja/index/).
[a] Department of Cardiology, Keio University School of Medicine, 35 Shinanomachi, Shinjuku, Tokyo 160-8582, Japan; [b] Department of Cardiology, Sakakibara Heart Institute, 3-16-1 Asahicho, Fuchu, Tokyo 183-0003, Japan; [c] Department of Cardiology, Saitama Medical University, International Medical Center, 1397-1 Yamane, Hidaka, Saitama 350-1298, Japan; [d] Department of Cardiology, National Defense Medical College, 3-2 Namiki-cho, Tokorozawa, Saitama 359-8513, Japan; [e] Department of Cardiovascular Medicine, Kyorin University School of Medicine, 6-20-2 Shinkawa, Mitaka, Tokyo 192-8508, Japan
* Corresponding author. Department of Cardiology, Keio University School of Medicine, 35 Shinanomachi Shinjuku-ku, Tokyo 160-8582, Japan.
E-mail address: sk@keio.jp

Cardiol Clin 39 (2021) 255–265
https://doi.org/10.1016/j.ccl.2021.01.008

treatment for patients with HF and a reduced ejection fraction (HFrEF), including patients with FMR. The American Heart Association/American College of Cardiology guidelines indicate that guideline-directed medical therapy (GDMT) is the first-line therapy for HFrEF and FMR, and the only Class I indication for treating FMR.[4] More recent large-scale randomized controlled trials have also indicated that sodium-glucose co-transporter-2 (SGLT2) inhibitors may help to decrease the risk of HF hospitalization and mortality.[5,6]

This review aims to cover the role of drug therapy and its optimization in the contemporary era for treating severe FMR.

GUIDELINE-DIRECTED MEDICAL THERAPY IN CLASSIC HEART FAILURE STUDIES

Neurohormonal antagonists can be prescribed to reduce morbidity and mortality among patients with HFrEF (**Table 1**). These drugs lead to a reduction in the left ventricular end-diastolic volume (LVEDV), which can be expected to reduce FMR if the degree of FMR is proportionate to the LVEDV. However, it is unclear whether the response of FMR to GDMT is an independent predictor of a favorable prognosis. Clinical trials of neurohormonal antagonists (usually in combination with loop diuretics) for HFrEF have typically not evaluated FMR severity before and after treatment, and the evidence to support pharmacologic interventions for FMR is derived from small-scale studies.

Treatment using angiotensin-converting enzyme inhibitors (ACEIs)/ angiotensin receptor blockers (ARBs) decreases the degree of FMR, typically in patients with mild-to-moderate MR. A high dose is usually required to achieve this benefit, and high doses are often specifically prescribed to patients who have a higher pretreatment LVEDV. A randomized trial evaluated 28 ambulatory patients with systolic ischemic HF (New York Heart Association functional class II–III; mean LVEF of 29%) who had grade 2 or higher FMR (>5 cm^2 regurgitation area on color flow Doppler ultrasound examination). The mitral regurgitation area decreased from the baseline value after the patient received a dose of 50 mg/d (3.1 cm^2), with a further decrease at a dose of 100 mg/d (5.3 cm^2), and these findings were associated with an increased forward stroke volume.[7]

Beta-blockers are also efficient for ameliorating FMR in patients with ischemic and nonischemic HF. For example, 1 study of 257 patients with chronic HF and LV systolic dysfunction revealed that carvedilol decreased the LVEDV and FMR severity (28% of patients had lower grade FMR after 24 months of treatment), with the extent of reverse ventricular remodeling being inversely related to the baseline degree of LV dilatation and independent of FMR or its severity.[8] Another study of severe MR evaluated 45 consecutive patients with chronic ischemic and nonischemic HF, who received carvedilol and were matched to a control group. After 6 months of carvedilol treatment, the LVEF had increased from 24% to 29%, which was associated with a significant reduction in the mitral regurgitant volume (50 mL/min vs 16 mL/min) that was not observed in the control group (57 mL/min vs 47 mL/min).[9]

A more recent study of 163 consecutive patients with HFrEF (LVEF of <40%) and grade 3 to 4+ FMR receiving maximally tolerated neurohormonal antagonists demonstrated that 38% of the 50 patients with severe FMR at baseline improved to nonsevere FMR, and 18% of the patients with nonsevere FMR at baseline progressed to severe FMR (median follow-up period of 50 months). Patients with sustained severe FMR or worsening of FMR had a 13% increase in their LVEDV index, and patients who experienced an improvement in their severe FMR had a 2% decrease in their LVEDV index.[10] Moreover, severe FMR was the most important independent predictor of major adverse cardiac events (a composite of all-cause death

---

Table 1
The drug agents listed in the clinical practice guidelines (guideline-directed medical therapy) for HF and their proven effects

Drug Agent	Proven Effect
Beta-blockers	Decrease the risks of HF hospitalization and mortality
ACEIs or ARBs	Decrease the risks of HF hospitalization and mortality
Angiotensin receptor neprilysin inhibitors to replace ACEIs or ARBs	Decrease the risks of HF hospitalization and mortality
Mineralocorticoid receptor antagonists	Decrease the risk of mortality
Ivabradine	Decrease the risk of HF hospitalization

Abbreviations: ACEI, angiotensin-converting enzyme inhibitors; ARB, angiotensin receptor blockers.

and heart transplantation or hospitalization for HF and/or malignant arrhythmias), regardless of sustained or worsening FMR status, with an adjusted odds ratio of 2.5 (95% confidence interval, 1.5–4.3).[10]

Among the studies described, FMR improvement was observed in less than one-half of the treated population.[7–10] Thus, it is important to consider whether it is possible to achieve earlier identification of patients who will not respond to medical therapy or who will develop more severe FMR. The increasing complexity of FMR treatment among patients with HF also highlights the need to achieve earlier and more frequent referrals to centers with expertise in treating these patients. Thus, early involvement of HF teams is essential for rapid treatment optimization in patients with FMR and HF, because other interventions might be possible if medical therapy fails, depending on the patient's condition.

Interestingly, patients who do not experience an improvement in MR severity after medical therapy have a high incidence of left bundle branch block.[10] Thus, in addition to pharmacologic management, cardiac resynchronization therapy (CRT) can also facilitate LV reverse remodeling and decrease FMR, especially in patients with ventricular dyssynchrony.[11] A study of 24 patients with HF with left bundle branch block revealed that CRT was associated with a 50% decrease in the effective regurgitant orifice area (EROA; from 25 mm^2 to 13 mm^2) during the acute phase of HF treatment.[12] Longer term beneficial effects have also been identified in large-scale randomized trials, such as the Multicenter InSync Randomized Clinical Evaluation (MIRACLE) trial, in which CRT produced significant reductions in the LV end-systolic and end-diastolic dimensions and the mitral regurgitant jet area (−2.7 cm^2 [CRT] vs −0.5 cm^2 [control] at 6 months).[13] The detailed effects of CRT on moderate-to-severe FMR were evaluated in a study of 98 consecutive patients who underwent CRT according to the current guidelines,[11] in which a significant improvement (reduction by at least 1 severity grade) was observed in 49% of patients. The survival rate was higher among patients with MR improvement, relative to among patients without MR improvement, and MR improvement was an independent prognostic factor (hazard ratio, 0.35; 95% confidence interval, 0.13–0.94).[11]

These findings highlight the importance of care when selecting CRT treatment for patients with FMR. A lack of response to CRT may be related to an inability to pace scarred regions, especially in patients with ischemic MR. The reported independent predictors of FMR reduction after CRT include anteroseptal to posterior wall radial strain dyssynchrony (>200 ms), an end-systolic dimension index of less than 29 mm/m^2, and lack of scarring at the papillary muscle insertion.[14]

GUIDELINE-DIRECTED MEDICAL THERAPY IN SURGICAL STUDIES

The surgical treatment of isolated FMR is associated with improvements in symptoms, quality of life, and reverse LV remodeling. However, its effects on FMR with LV dysfunction remains controversial, because the prognosis of FMR is mainly associated with LV dysfunction and its etiology.[15] Surgical intervention for FMR has been evaluated in randomized controlled trials conducted by the Cardiothoracic Surgical Trials Network, which revealed that mitral valve repair was associated with a significantly higher rate of recurrent moderate or severe MR at 2 years (58%), relative to mitral valve replacement (3.8%). Although the 30-day mortality rate tended to be higher in the replacement group (4.0% vs 1.6%), there were no significant differences in the rates of all-cause mortality and major adverse cardiac or cerebrovascular events at 2 years.[16] The second Cardiothoracic Surgical Trials Network trial compared coronary artery bypass grafting (CABG) alone to CABG plus mitral valve repair in 301 patients with coronary artery disease and moderate FMR. Moderate or severe MR was significantly more common in the CABG group (32.3%) than in the CABG plus mitral repair group (11.2%), although the 2 groups had similar rates of all-cause mortality, major adverse cardiac or cerebrovascular events, readmission, and cardiovascular readmission.[17]

To date, no studies have shown that mitral valve surgery improves survival in FMR cases, relative to GDMT alone.[18–22] However, no surgical studies have required medical therapy to be optimized by HF specialists. One study evaluated whether mitral valve annuloplasty or HF medications influenced mortality among patients with FMR and LV dysfunction using propensity score matching analysis. That study revealed no demonstrable change in mortality after annuloplasty, although reduced risks of mortality were associated with treatment using ACEIs (hazard ratio, 0.65; 95% confidence interval, 0.44–0.95) or beta-blockers (hazard ratio, 0.59; 95% confidence interval, 0.42–0.83), and a significantly increased risk of mortality was associated with digoxin treatment (hazard ratio, 1.66; 95% confidence interval, 1.15–2.39).[23] The Effectiveness of Surgical Mitral Valve Repair versus Medical Treatment for People with Significant Mitral Regurgitation and Nonischemic Congestive Heart Failure trial (SMMART-HF, NCT0068140) was designed to compare the safety and effectiveness of GDMT with or without surgical mitral annuloplasty for nonischemic patients with HF with FMR, although the trial was terminated early owing to inadequate enrollment. A similar patient population was tested in the Cardiovascular Outcomes Assessment of the Mitra-Clip Percutaneous Therapy for Heart Failure Patients with Functional MR trial (COAPT). Therefore, the current guideline recommendations for mitral valve surgery as FMR treatment are more conservative than for other therapeutic options. According to the 2020 Focused Update of the American College of Cardiology Expert Consensus Decision Pathway, mitral valve surgery (either replacement or repair) is considered reasonable at the time of other cardiac surgery and can be considered as an isolated procedure for select patients with advanced New York Heart Association functional class, despite guideline-directed management including CRT when indicated.[24] In addition, patients who do not respond to CRT may be considered for transcatheter mitral valve repair using the MitraClip device if the anatomic findings are appropriate and the procedure is selected by a multidisciplinary heart team.

The main determinants of surgical failure to treat FMR might be related to the heterogeneity of the patients who were included in the clinical trials, and it is unclear whether more advanced surgical techniques and/or better patient selection might improve outcomes. For example, atrial FMR (FMR solely owing to annular dilation) is a distinct clinical form of FMR only recently recognized. Its prevalence and efficacy of surgical and medical therapy is still scarcely investigated, although small-scale studies have shown a possible benefit of ARB to leaflet remodeling in patients with atrial FMR, the entity is still under-recognized and under-reported.[25]

The trials listed in the present section typically included a broad range of patients with MR based on annular dilation, multiple jets, advanced ventricular remodeling, excessive tethering, end-systolic interpapillary muscle distance, and systolic sphericity index. A recent meta-analysis revealed that mitral valve repair is associated with lower operative mortality than valve replacement in patients with ischemic MR.[26] This finding also agrees with evidence from the first Cardiothoracic Surgical Trials Network trial that suggested that repair tended to produce better perioperative survival, although the 30-day mortality rate was almost 3-fold higher, which is likely because that study was not powered to evaluate 30-day mortality.[16]

GUIDELINE-DIRECTED MEDICAL THERAPY IN MitraClip STUDIES

The MITRA-FR trial was a multicenter, randomized, open-label clinical trial of transcatheter mitral valve repair using the MitraClip, which was compared with medical therapy among symptomatic French patients with FMR. The key inclusion criteria were severe MR (EROA of >20 mm^2 or a regurgitant volume of >30 mL/beat), an EF of 15% to 40%, at least one HF-related hospitalization during the previous year, and ineligibility for surgery. Medical therapy was optimized by local investigators and most patients were receiving loop diuretics, beta-blockers, and ACEIs, ARBs, or angiotensin receptor neprilysin inhibitors (ARNIs). The rates of CRT were 30% in the Mitra-Clip arm and 23% in the control arm.[27]

The COAPT trial was an American multicenter randomized controlled trial that compared the MitraClip and GDMT with GDMT alone for patients with symptomatic moderately severe or severe MR. The key inclusion criteria were moderately severe (3+) or severe (4+) MR confirmed by a core echocardiography laboratory, an EF of 20% to 50%, an LVEDV of 70 mL or less, at least 1 HF-related hospitalization during the last year, and/or an elevated B-type natriuretic peptide concentration (>300 pg/mL adjusted for body mass index), and not a candidate for mitral valve surgery at the enrolling center. A central eligibility committee confirmed that all patients fulfilled the enrollment criteria (including the use of maximal GDMT doses).[28]

Both trials included high and very similar proportions of patients who were receiving GDMT at baseline. The baseline use of renin–angiotensin system inhibitors was higher in the MITRA-FR trial (mean, 73.7%; device arm, 73.0%; control arm, 74.3%) than in the COAPT trial (mean, 67.1%; device arm, 71.5%; control arm, 62.8%). Furthermore, more patients in the MITRA-FR trial received a combination of renin–angiotensin system inhibitors and ARNIs (11.1% vs 3.6%). However, similar rates of beta-blocker use were observed in the MITRA-FR trial (mean, 89.5%; device arm, 88.2%; control arm, 90.8%) and in the COAPT trial (mean, 90.4%; device arm, 91.1%; control arm, 89.7%).

The discrepancy in the results of these 2 trials might be related to only the COAPT trial requiring patients to use maximally tolerated GDMT before enrollment. In addition, it is not clear what proportion of patients in the COAPT trial were receiving target doses of the recommended drugs or had blood pressure levels that would have prohibited further dose titration. Nevertheless, the device arm of the COAPT trial had a significantly higher beta-blocker dose, relative to the control arm. Furthermore, blood pressure levels increased after the MitraClip procedure and allowed for further treatment optimization in the device arm (increase dose by >100% or new drug class started: 8.6% in the device arm and 3.8% in the control arm; $P = .01$). Thus, patients who undergo transcatheter mitral valve repair using the MitraClip might be able to tolerate higher GDMT doses that were not previously tolerated.[29]

MEDICAL THERAPY IN PROPORTIONATE AND DISPROPORTIONATE MITRAL REGURGITATION

The patients in the COAPT trial had MR severity that was disproportionate to their LV remodeling, whereas patients in the MITRA-FR trial had larger LV volumes and less severe MR.[30] The difference in the prevalences of proportionate and disproportionate MR is widely thought to be related to different definitions of MR severity that are used in the American and European clinical practice guidelines. For example, the 2017 American guidelines characterize MR severity according to the magnitude of regurgitant flow, with severe MR identified based on a regurgitant fraction of 50% or greater, a regurgitant volume of 60 mL or greater, or an EROA of 40 mm^2 or greater.[4] In contrast, the European guidelines determined the severity of MR based on prognosis; patients with an EROA higher than 20 mm^2 are known to have a mortality risk compared with those with normal EROA values, severe MR was considered present for all patients with an EROA of 20 mm^2 or greater.[31] It is noteworthy that many of these patients with MR might have had their prognosis determined by the severity of LV dysfunction, rather than MR.

The COAPT trial protocol required all patients to be receiving maximally tolerated GDMT, which might have promoted the inclusion of patients with disproportionate MR. For example, patients with proportionate MR might have responded favorably to GDMT (based on the regurgitant flow magnitude) and thus been excluded from the COAPT trial. In contrast, the MITRA-FR trial participants seemed to have a higher likelihood of proportionate MR based on the echocardiographic inclusion criteria (eg, low EROA criteria without a designated upper limit for LV volumetry). In this context, it might be difficult to achieve and maintain coaptation of the valve leaflets using mechanical clips for a markedly dilated LV that remains dilated during long-term follow-up (as in the MITRA-FR trial).[29] Thus, based on the distinction between proportionate and disproportionate MR, recent reviews and commentaries have suggested that medical therapy should be directed primarily at improving LV function in patients with proportionate MR. If LV dilatation explains the degree of MR, treatments that lead to reversal of LV remodeling can decrease the degree of MR and thus decrease morbidity and mortality. In contrast, patients with disproportionate MR should undergo interventions that are directed toward the mitral valve apparatus (including the annulus, chordae, and papillary muscles). In these patients, drugs that decrease the LV volume would not be expected to ameliorate the MR, which might respond only to treatments that restore the integrity of the leaflets or supporting structures. **Table 2** includes a summary of the findings from related studies.

The MITRA-FR and COAPT trials revealed that amelioration of functional MR might be achieved using ACEIs, ARBs, beta-blockers, and ARNIs.[27,28] Patients whose MR responds favorably to these drugs have the largest pretreatment LVEDV,[32] whereas patients with disproportionate MR do not respond favorably to medical therapy.[28] The presence of a left bundle branch block is a principal factor that is associated with MR nonresponse to neurohormonal antagonists.[10,28] Later subsets of patients (defined based on the degree of regurgitation, degree of LV remodeling/dysfunction, or the combination of these parameters) from the MITRA-FR trial were evaluated to identify patients that might benefit from percutaneous repair or medical therapy alone.[27,33] However, in both the intention-to-treat and per-protocol analyses, there were no significant interactions between the trial group and any of those subsets in terms of a composite outcome involving all-cause death or unplanned hospitalization for HF at 24 months. Nevertheless, it should be noted that the most disproportionate subset was defined as an EROA 30 mm^2 or greater and an LVEDV of less than 242 mL. Bartko and colleagues[34] recently characterized the prognostic importance of proportionate and disproportionate MR among 291 patients with functional MR and LV systolic dysfunction. In that study, patients with disproportionate functional MR had a nearly 2-fold increase in mortality, although it is interesting that similar survivals were observed for patients with severe proportionate MR and patients with nonsevere MR. Therefore, it is possible that patients with proportionate MR might respond favorably to GDMT, whereas patients with disproportionate MR might not, although further studies are needed to validate this attractive concept in the clinical setting.

ROLE OF NOVEL HEART FAILURE AGENTS

Recent clinical evidence has identified benefits in cases of HFrEF after treatment using some novel

Table 2
GDMT for proportionate and disproportionate functional moderate-to-severe mitral regurgitation

Cohort	Proportionate or Disproportionate	GDMT	LVEF	LVEDV	EROA	Effect on MR	Effect on clinical Events	Ref.
COAPT (control arm)	Disproportionate	Anti-HF therapy using loop diuretics (89%), beta-blockers (90%), ACEIs (27%), ARBs (23%), and ARNIs (3%), according to the 2017 AHA guidelines.[31] The therapy was maximized at the time of enrollment and optimized by a heart team, which included HF specialists, during follow-up (control arm only).	30	191 ± 73	40 ± 15	Decreased, but less effective than the Mitra-Clip arm (reduction of MR ≤2: 40% vs 87% at 12 mo)	Less effective than the Mitra-Clip arm (composite outcome: 66% vs 45% at 24 mo)	Stone et al,[28] 2018
MITRA-FR (control arm)	Proportionate	Pre-enrollment anti-HF therapy using loop diuretics (98%), beta-blockers (91%), ACEI/ARB (74%), and ARNI (12%), according to the 2016 ESC guidelines.[32] Therapy was optimized by local investigators (control arm only).	33	250 ± 75	31 ± 11	Unchanged and less effective than the Mitra-Clip arm (ΔRV: −4 mL vs −24 mL at 12 mo)	Comparable with the Mitra-Clip arm (composite outcome: 51% vs 57% at 12 mo)	Obadia et al,[27] 2018

Trial	MR type	Pre-enrollment therapy	N	LVEDV	EROA			Outcome	Reference
MITRA-FR (subgroup in control arm)	Equivocal or disproportionate	Pre-enrollment anti-HF therapy using loop diuretics (98%), beta-blockers (91%), ACEI/ARB (74%), and ARNI (12%), according to the 2016 ESC guidelines.[32] Therapy was optimized by local investigators (control arm only).	33 (control arm only)	<242	≥30	N/A		Comparable with the Mitra-Clip arm (composite outcome: 63% vs 48% at 24 mo)	Bartko et al,[34] 2019
Severe MR	Disproportionate (if LBBB)	Anti-HF therapy using loop diuretics (86%), beta-blockers (94%), and ACEI/ARBs (76%).	27	~200	N/A	N/A	Decrease from severe to nonsevere MR	Mortality rate of ~20% at 56 mo	Nasser et al,[10] 2017
Severe MR	Disproportionate	Anti-HF therapy using ACEI/ARBs (93%), beta-blockers (86%), and MRAs (63%).	25 (total)	~200	~30	N/A		Less effective than the proportionate group (mortality rate: 50% vs 25% at 80 mo)	McMurray et al,[35] 2014

Abbreviations: ACEI, angiotensin-converting enzyme inhibitor; AHA, American Heart Association; ARB, angiotensin receptor blocker; ARNI, angiotensin receptor neprilysin inhibitor; EROA, effective regurgitant orifice area; ESC, European Society of Cardiology; LBBB, left bundle branch block; LVEDV, left ventricular end-diastolic volume; LVEF, left ventricular ejection fraction; MR, mitral regurgitation; MRA, mineralocorticoid receptor antagonist; N/A, not applicable.

agents in addition to GDMT (ACEIs, ARBs, beta-blockers, and mineralocorticoid receptor antagonists). However, there are few data regarding the effects of these agents on cardiac structure, cardiac function, and FMR.

Sacubitril/valsartan is an ARNI that is associated with a decrease (vs enalapril) in clinical adverse events, such as cardiovascular death or hospitalization for acute HF, among patients with HFrEF.[35] Some studies have identified reverse LV remodeling after ARNI administration,[36–38] and one of those studies revealed that a decrease in MR was associated with an improved LVEF and a decreased LV volume.[37] Kang and colleagues[39] performed a multicenter prospective study of patients with HFrEF who were randomized to receive sacubitril/valsartan or valsartan, and evaluated the longitudinal change in FMR as a primary end point. At 12 months after randomization, the sacubitril/valsartan group had significant decreases in the EROA and regurgitant volume, although the lack of a significant difference in blood pressure between the 2 groups suggests that the effects of sacubitril/valsartan on FMR were not related to reduced afterload.

Improved clinical outcomes can also be observed after treatment using SGLT2 inhibitors, such as empagliflozin[6] and dapagliflozin,[5] especially in terms of the acute HF hospitalization rate, regardless of whether the patient has diabetes.[5,6] These agents also consistently provide a decrease in LV mass and an improvement in LV diastolic function (represented by E/e' and left atrial volume) in patients with diabetes.[40–42] Nevertheless, other studies revealed only a modest improvement in LVEF after SGLT2 inhibitor treatment for patients with HF,[40,43] and these drugs' effects on LV systolic function or geometry remain controversial.[42,44–46] One study used MRI to compare cardiac geometry between patients who received SGLT2 inhibitors or a placebo, and revealed that SGLT2 inhibitors did not produce any noticeable change in cardiac geometry.[46] However, those studies only evaluated small samples of patients (n < 100) and did not directly evaluate whether SGLT2 inhibitors influenced FMR. Thus, further large-scale studies are needed to determine whether SGLT2 inhibitors can influence FMR in patients with HF.

Vericiguat is a soluble guanylate cyclase stimulator that was shown to decrease the incidences of cardiovascular death or HF hospitalization among patients with HFrEF.[47] A phase II trial also revealed that vericiguat provided a marginal increase in LVEF, but did not influence LV volume.[48] No reports have described its effects on other echocardiographic parameters, including FMR.

REGIONAL DIFFERENCES IN HEART FAILURE CARE

Among patients with chronic HF, numerous studies have identified substantial regional variations in the patterns of GDMT prescriptions for patients with HFrEF.[49–51] A report from the National Cardiovascular Registry Practice Innovation and Clinical Excellence (PINNACLE) evaluated 40 American cardiology institutions and revealed substantial variability in the use of ACEIs/ARBs (44%–100%) and beta-blockers (49%–100%).[49] A study of an international registry that included 547 centers in 36 countries from Africa, Asia, Australia, Europe, the Middle East, and the Americas revealed globally satisfactory adherence to GDMT for HFrEF, albeit with low adherence in some regions, particularly in Central and Eastern Europe.[50] The latest report from the multinational ASIAN-HF registry, which included 46 centers in 11 Asian countries, revealed that physicians in high-income countries (eg, Singapore, Hong Kong, Korea, and Japan) were more likely to prescribe the guideline-recommended combination of ACEIs/ARBs and beta-blocker therapies, relative to physicians in the low-income countries.[51] Furthermore, that study revealed regional variations in using the guideline-recommended doses and the mean doses that were achieved during GDMT therapy. Interestingly, Japan had the second highest use of beta-blockers (91%) but the lowest achieved dose, with 41% of patients receiving less than 25% of the guideline-recommended dose. These variations in prescription patterns are likely related to several factors: (1) differences in patient age, frailty, and comorbidities, (2) physician tendency to focus on symptom relief, rather than mortality reduction, as well as under-recognition of the importance of GDMT, and (3) treatment costs or access to medical care. There is also significant variability in the etiologic factors, precipitants, and points of hospital entry in cases of acute HF.[52] Finally, the difference may reflect variations in treatment algorithms, a lack of guideline implementation, local medication availability, variability in regional practice patterns, or difficulty in generalizing clinical trial data to different regions of the world.

Maggioni and colleagues[53] have demonstrated that patients with MR are likely to receive inappropriate GDMT. However, to date, no studies have identified regional variations in GDMT among patients with HF and severe FMR. Given that patients with HFrEF with severe FMR are generally older, frail, and have comorbidities,[28,54] physicians may be less likely to optimize GDMT and may instead emphasize symptom relief over a decrease in the risk of mortality.[55] Thus, it is plausible that similar regional variations exist in the optimization of GDMT among patients with severe FMR. Research is needed to identify barriers to implementing the recommended GDMT and learning from practice patterns in other regions, which may help to improve the quality of medical management and outcomes for patients with HFrEF with FMR.

SUMMARY

Baseline GDMT remains the cornerstone of treatment for FMR when considering surgical or transcatheter treatments. Early involvement of clinical teams including physicians who are familiar with GDMT is essential for the rapid treatment optimization in patients with FMR and HF. Surgical and percutaneous interventions would become valid options if medical therapy fails after thorough investigation of patient's overall condition. However, systematic evaluation on the effect of GDMT in broader spectrum of FMR outside of substudies from recent clinical trials (eg, MITRA-FR or COAPT) is lacking. Future clinical studies, with well-structured clinical and echocardiographic variables with their serial assessment, along with implementation of GDMT (including novel HF agents) are needed.

CLINICS CARE POINTS

- Guideline-directed medical therapy remains the mainstay of treatment for patients with functional mitral regurgitation.

- This review revisits the role of medical therapy and its optimization for severe functional mitral regurgitation.

REFERENCES

1. Benjamin EJ, Muntner P, Alonso A, et al. Heart disease and stroke statistics – 2019 update: a report from the American Heart Association. Circulation 2019;139:e56–528.
2. de Marchena E, Badiye A, Robalino G, et al. Prevalence of the different Carpentier classes of mitral regurgitation: a stepping stone for future therapeutic research and development. J Card Surg 2011;26: 385–92.
3. Sannino A, Smith RL, Schiattarella GG, et al. Survival and cardiovascular outcomes of patients with secondary mitral regurgitation: a systematic review and meta-analysis. JAMA Cardiol 2017;2:1130–9.
4. Nishimura RA, Otto CM, Bonow RO, et al. 2017 AHA/ACC focused update of the 2014 AHA/ACC guideline for the management of patients with valvular heart disease: a report of the American College of Cardiology/American Heart Association Task Force on clinical practice guidelines. Circulation 2017; 135:e1159–95.
5. McMurray JJV, Solomon SD, Inzucchi SE, et al. Dapagliflozin in patients with heart failure and reduced ejection fraction. N Engl J Med 2019;381: 1995–2008.
6. Packer M, Anker SD, Butler J, et al. Cardiovascular and renal outcomes with empagliflozin in HF. N Engl J Med 2020. https://doi.org/10.1056/NEJMoa2022190.
7. Seneviratne B, Moore GA, West PD. Effect of captopril on functional mitral regurgitation in dilated heart failure: a randomised double blind placebo controlled trial. Br Heart J 1994;72:63–8.
8. Kotlyar E, Hayward CS, Keogh AM, et al. The impact of baseline left ventricular size and mitral regurgitation on reverse left ventricular remodeling in response to carvedilol: size does not matter. Heart 2004;90:800–1.
9. Capomolla S, Febo O, Gnemmi M, et al. Beta-blockade therapy in chronic heart failure: diastolic function and mitral regurgitation improvement by carvedilol. Am Heart J 2000;139:596–608.
10. Nasser R, Van Assche L, Vorlat A, et al. Evolution of functional mitral regurgitation and prognosis in medically managed heart failure patients with reduced ejection fraction. JACC Heart Fail 2017;5: 652–9.
11. van Bommel RJ, Marsan NA, Delgado V, et al. Cardiac resynchronization therapy is a therapeutic option in patients with moderate-to-severe functional mitral regurgitation and high operative risk. Circulation 2011;124:912–9.
12. Breithardt OA, Sinha AM, Schwammenthal E, et al. Acute effects of cardiac resynchronization therapy on functional mitral regurgitation in patients with advanced systolic heart failure. J Am Coll Cardiol 2003;41:765–70.
13. Abraham WT, Fisher WG, Smith AL, et al. Cardiac resynchronization in chronic heart failure. N Engl J Med 2002;346:1845–53.
14. Onishi T, Onishi T, Marek JJ, et al. Mechanistic features associated with improvement in mitral regurgitation after cardiac resynchronization therapy and their relation to long-term patient outcomes. Circ Heart Fail 2013;6:685–93.
15. De Bonis M, Lapenna E, Verzini A, et al. The recurrence of mitral regurgitation parallels the absence of left ventricular reverse remodeling after mitral

repair in patients with advanced dilated cardiomyopathy. Ann Thorac Surg 2008;85(3):932–9.

16. Goldstein D, Moskowitz AJ, Gelijns AC, et al. Two-year outcomes of surgical treatment of severe ischemic mitral regurgitation. N Engl J Med 2016; 374:344–53.

17. Michler RE, Smith PK, Parides MK, et al. Two-year outcomes of surgical treatment of moderate ischemic mitral regurgitation. N Engl J Med 2016; 374:1932–41.

18. Bolling SF, Pagani FD, Deeb GM, et al. Intermediate-term outcome of mitral reconstruction in cardiomyopathy. J Thorac Cardiovasc Surg 1998;115:381–8.

19. Rothenburger M, Rukosujew A, Hammel D, et al. Mitral valve surgery in patients with poor left ventricular function. Thorac Cardiovasc Surg 2002;50(6):351–4.

20. Gummert JF, Rahmel A, Bucerius J, et al. Mitral valve repair in patients with end-stage cardiomyopathy: who benefits? Eur J Cardiothorac Surg 2003;23(6): 1017–22.

21. Bishay ES, McCarthy PM, Cosgrove DM, et al. Mitral valve surgery in patients with severe left ventricular dysfunction. Eur J Cardiothorac Surg 2000;17: 213–21.

22. Chen FY, Adams DH, Aranki SF, et al. Mitral valve repair in cardiomyopathy. Circulation 1998;98: II124–7.

23. Wu AH, Aaronson KD, Bolling SF, et al. Impact of mitral valve annuloplasty on mortality risk in patients with mitral regurgitation and left ventricular systolic dysfunction. J Am Coll Cardiol 2005;45(3):381–7.

24. Bonow RO, O'Gara PT, Adams DH, et al. 2020 focused update of the 2017 ACC Expert Consensus Decision Pathway on the management of mitral regurgitation: a report of the American College of cardiology Solution Set Oversight committee. J Am Coll Cardiol 2020;75(17):2236–70.

25. Deferm S, Bertrand PB, Verbrugge FH, et al. Atrial functional mitral regurgitation: JACC review topic of the week. J Am Coll Cardiol 2019;73(19):2465–76.

26. Dayan V, Soca G, Cura L, et al. Similar survival after mitral valve replacement or repair for ischemic mitral regurgitation: a meta-analysis. Ann Thorac Surg 2014;97(3):758–65.

27. Obadia JF, Messika-Zeitoun D, Leurent G, et al. Percutaneous repair or medical treatment for secondary mitral regurgitation. N Engl J Med 2018; 379:2297–306.

28. Stone GW, Lindenfeld J, Abraham WT, et al. Transcatheter mitral valve repair in patients with heart failure. N Engl J Med 2018;379:2307–18.

29. Grayburn PA, Sannino A, Packer M. Proportionate and disproportionate functional mitral regurgitation: a new conceptual framework that reconciles the results of the MITRA-FR and COAPT Trials. JACC Cardiovasc Imaging 2019;12:353–62.

30. Packer M, Grayburn PA. New evidence supporting a novel conceptual framework for distinguishing proportionate and disproportionate functional mitral regurgitation. JAMA Cardiol 2020;5:469–75.

31. Ponikowski P, Voors AA, Anker SD, et al. 2016 ESC Guidelines for the diagnosis and treatment of acute and chronic heart failure: the Task Force for the diagnosis and treatment of acute and chronic heart failure of the European Society of Cardiology (ESC) developed with the special contribution of the Heart Failure Association (HFA) of the ESC. Eur Heart J 2016;37:2129–200.

32. Packer M, Grayburn PA. Contrasting effects of pharmacological, procedural, and surgical interventions on proportionate and disproportionate functional mitral regurgitation in chronic heart failure. Circulation 2019;140:779–89.

33. Messika-Zeitoun D, Iung B, Armoiry X, et al. Impact of mitral regurgitation severity and left ventricular remodeling on outcomes after Mitraclip implantation: results from the Mitra-FR trial. JACC Cardiovasc Imaging 2020. https://doi.org/10.1016/j.jcmg.2020.07. 021. S1936-878X;30645–8.

34. Bartko PE, Heitzinger G, Arfsten H, et al. Disproportionate functional mitral regurgitation: advancing a conceptual framework to clinical practice. JACC Cardiovasc Imaging 2019;12:2088–90.

35. McMurray JJ, Packer M, Desai AS, et al. Angiotensin-neprilysin inhibition versus enalapril in heart failure. N Engl J Med 2014;371:993–1004.

36. Almufleh A, Marbach J, Chih S, et al. Ejection fraction improvement and reverse remodeling achieved with sacubitril/valsartan in patients with heart failure with reduced ejection fraction. Am J Cardiovasc Dis 2017;7:108–13.

37. Martens P, Beliën H, Dupont M, et al. The reverse remodeling response to sacubitril/valsartan therapy in heart failure with reduced ejection fraction. Cardiovasc Ther 2018;36:e12435.

38. Bayard G, Da Costa A, Pierrard R, et al. Impact of sacubitril/valsartan on echo parameters in heart failure patients with reduced ejection fraction: a prospective evaluation. Int J Cardiol Heart Vasc 2019; 25:100418.

39. Kang DH, Park SJ, Shin SH, et al. Angiotensin receptor inhibitor neprilysin inhibitor for functional mitral regurgitation. Circulation 2019;139:1354–65.

40. Soga F, Tanaka H, Tatsumi K, et al. Impact of dapagliflozin on left ventricular diastolic function in patients with type 2 diabetes mellitus with chronic heart failure. Cardiovasc Diabetol 2018;17:132.

41. Matsutani D, Sakamoto M, Kayama Y, et al. Effect of canagliflozin on left ventricular diastolic function in patients with type 2 diabetes. Cardiovasc Diabetol 2018;17:73.

42. Zhang DP, Xu L, Wang LF, et al. Effects of antidiabetic drugs on left ventricular function/dysfunction:

a systematic review and network meta-analysis. Cardiovasc Diabetol 2020;19:10.

43. Tanaka H, Soga F, Tatsumi K, et al. Positive effect of dapagliflozin on left ventricular longitudinal function in patients with type 2 diabetes mellitus and chronic heart failure. Cardiovasc Diabetol 2020;19:6.

44. Bonora BM, Vigili de Kreutzenberg S, Avogaro A, et al. Effects of the SGLT2 inhibitor dapagliflozin on cardiac function evaluated by impedance cardiography in patients with type 2 diabetes. Secondary analysis of a randomized placebo-controlled trial. Cardiovasc Diabetol 2019;18:106.

45. Hsu JC, Wang CY, Su MM, et al. Effect of empagliflozin on cardiac function, adiposity, and diffuse fibrosis in patients with type 2 diabetes mellitus. Sci Rep 2019;9:15348.

46. Singh JSS, Mordi IR, Vickneson K, et al. Dapagliflozin versus placebo on left ventricular remodeling in patients with diabetes and heart failure: the REFORM trial. Diabetes Care 2020;43:1356–9.

47. Armstrong PW, Pieske B, Anstrom KJ, et al. Vericiguat in patients with heart failure and reduced ejection fraction. N Engl J Med 2020;382:1883–93.

48. Gheorghiade M, Greene SJ, Butler J, et al. Effect of vericiguat, a soluble guanylate cyclase stimulator, on natriuretic peptide levels in patients with worsening chronic heart failure and reduced ejection fraction: the SOCRATES-REDUCED randomized trial. JAMA 2015;314:2251–62.

49. Peterson PN, Chan PS, Spertus JA, et al. Practice-level variation in use of recommended medications among outpatients with heart failure insights from the NCDR PINNACLE Program. Circ Heart Fail 2013;6:1132–8.

50. Komajda M, Anker SD, Cowie MR, et al. Physicians' adherence to guideline-recommended medications in heart failure with reduced ejection fraction: data from the QUALIFY global survey. Eur J Heart Fail 2016;18:514–22.

51. Teng THK, Tromp J, Tay WT, et al. Prescribing patterns of evidence-based heart failure pharmacotherapy and outcomes in the ASIAN-HF registry: a cohort study. Lancet Glob Heal 2018;6:e1008–18.

52. Filippatos G, Angermann CE, Cleland JGF, et al. Global differences in characteristics, precipitants, and initial management of patients presenting with acute heart failure. JAMA Cardiol 2020;5:401–10.

53. Maggioni AP, Van Gool K, Biondi N, et al. Appropriateness of prescriptions of recommended treatments in Organisation for Economic Co-operation and development health systems: findings based on the long-term registry of the European Society of cardiology on heart failure. Value Health 2015; 18:1098–104.

54. Maucort-Boulch D, Carrié D, Guerin P, et al. Percutaneous repair or medical treatment for secondary mitral regurgitation. N Engl J Med 2018;379: 2297–306.

55. Akita K, Kohno T, Kohsaka S, et al. Current use of guideline-based medical therapy in elderly patients admitted with acute heart failure with reduced ejection fraction and its impact on event-free survival. Int J Cardiol 2017;235:162–8.

Periprocedural Echocardiographic Guidance of Transcatheter Mitral Valve Edge-to-Edge Repair Using the MitraClip

Jay Ramchand, MBBS, BMedSci*, Rhonda Miyasaka, MD

KEYWORDS

- Mitral regurgitation • Echocardiography • Heart failure

KEY POINTS

- Transcatheter mitral valve repair using edge-to-edge clip has been established as an alternative to open surgical repair in primary and secondary mitral valve diseases.
- Optimal periprocedural imaging using transesophageal echocardiography is critical to determine procedural candidacy and ensure safe and successful implantation.
- Multiplanar reconstruction can be used to display all key mitral views, including the long axis, bicommissural, short axis, and 3-dimensional en face views.
- The use of this technique with and without color Doppler allows determination of MR mechanism and origin with precision.
- For optimal periprocedural imaging guidance, we recommend a detailed echocardiographic approach using the 7 steps outlined in this review article.

INTRODUCTION

In individuals with significantly increased surgical risk, a reduction of mitral regurgitation (MR) severity can be accomplished percutaneously by approximation of the anterior and posterior mitral leaflets, with transcatheter edge-to-edge mitral valve (MV) repair. The procedure is a percutaneous adaptation to the surgically performed Alfieri stitch and results in a double orifice valve (∞). Although the initial application of MitraClip was limited to patients with predominantly central MR and degenerative disease, recent clinical trials in addition to improved technical experience and advancements in 3-dimensional (3D) echocardiography has allowed successful application

to those with noncentral MR and secondary valve disease.[1]

Optimal periprocedural imaging using transesophageal echocardiography (TEE) is critical to determine procedural candidacy and ensure safe and successful implantation. In this review, we present a step by step overview of echocardiographic imaging for transcatheter MV edge-to-edge repair using the MitraClip device.

MITRAL VALVE ANATOMY

A comprehensive appreciation of MV anatomy and surrounding structures is important to facilitate optimal imaging guidance for transcatheter edge-to-edge MV repair. A detailed discussion of this

Department of Cardiovascular Medicine, Heart and Vascular Institute, Cleveland Clinic, 9500 Euclid Avenue, Cleveland, OH 44195, USA
* Corresponding author.
E-mail address: ramchaj@ccf.org

Cardiol Clin 39 (2021) 267–280
https://doi.org/10.1016/j.ccl.2021.01.009
0733-8651/21/© 2021 Elsevier Inc. All rights reserved.

is beyond the scope of this review and has been covered elsewhere.[2]

In brief, the MV complex comprises the mitral annulus, anterior and posterior leaflets, chordae tendinea, and papillary muscles (**Fig. 1**). The annulus marking the hinge line of the valvular leaflets is D shaped rather than circular.[3] The aortic valve is in fibrous continuity with the anterior leaflet of the MV. The annulus opposite the area of valvar fibrous continuity lacks a well-formed fibrous cord and tends to be weaker and hence more significantly affected in annular dilation.

OVERVIEW OF DEVICES AND PROCEDURE

The MitraClip device (Abbott Vascular, Menlo Park, CA) is a clip made of 2 polyester-covered arms roughly 8 mm long and 4 mm wide that functions to grasp both the anterior and posterior MV leaflets (**Fig. 2**). The clip is delivered by means of a 24F steerable catheter and triaxial delivery system via a femoral venous and transseptal approach to reach the systemic side and thus the MV.

The MitraClip NT_R and XT_R systems were introduced in 2018 and are an updated version of the previous versions of MitraClip (MitraClip and MitraClip NT). The XT_R device has 3 mm longer arms (with 2 extra rows of frictional elements), that expand the reach of the device by 5 mm compared with the MitraClip NT_R device. In general, the NT_R system is favored in patients with short, restricted leaflets (functional MR) or if there is concern for smaller MV area (MVA). The XT_R

device, is favored with degenerative MR with longer leaflet lengths, larger, wider flail width, and gaps. Indications and contraindications have previously been discussed elsewhere.[2,4]

MitraClip implantation is performed under general anesthesia owing to the need for a controlled environment that allows real-time and often prolonged TEE guidance. In addition, controlled breath holds can then be performed to maximize stability during leaflet grasping, a sensitive step of the procedure. In brief, after gaining transfemoral venous access, transseptal puncture (TSP) is performed to allow the MitraClip device to access the left atrium, where it is aligned with the mitral pathology, and then advanced into the left ventricle. The MitraClip system is then withdrawn toward the MV with the clip arms open and approximated to both the anterior and posterior leaflets. The grippers are then lowered to trap the leaflets between the grippers and the arms. Finally, the arms are then closed to oppose the anterior and posterior leaflets. If necessary, the device can be reopened for adjustment before device release and final deployment. Detailed echocardiographic evaluation is divided into 7 main steps which is covered step by step elsewhere in this article.

Procedural Guidance

Step 1: preprocedure evaluation
After the initiation of general anesthesia, TEE should be performed to complete a quick preprocedural checklist (**Table 1**). The first step is to

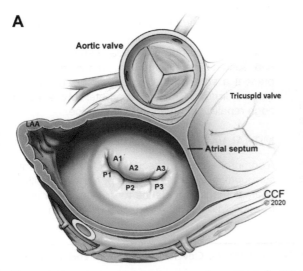
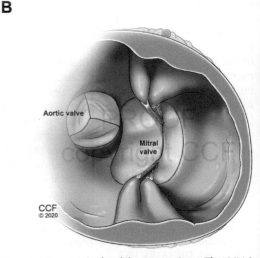

Fig. 1. MV anatomy. The MV as seen from the left atrial (*A*) and left ventricular (*B*) perspectives. The MV is composed of 2 leaflets, anterior and posterior, each of which is divided into 3 scallops, A1, A2, A3 and P1, P2, P3, as depicted. LAA, left atrial appendage. (Reprinted with permission, Cleveland Clinic Center for Medical Art & Photography ©2020. All Rights Reserved.)

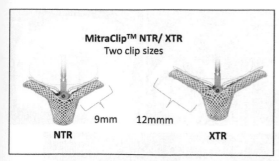

MitraClip™ NTR/ XTR
Two clip sizes

9mm   12mmm

NTR   XTR

Fig. 2. MitraClip devices. The MitraClip NT$_R$ and XT$_R$ systems introduced in 2018 comes in 2 sizes. The MitraClip XT$_R$ device has 3 mm longer arms that expand the reach of the device by 5 mm over that of the MitraClip NT$_R$ device. (Images courtesy of Abbott Vascular, Menlo Park, CA.)

confirm MR mechanism and origin to ensure there are no significant changes compared with prior imaging that would alter the plan for device placement. The pulmonary veins should be assessed to evaluate for flow reversal. Mitral stenosis should be assessed with the MVA and mean gradient. A MVA of less than 4.0 cm^2 is considered a relative contraindication to the procedure because deployment of the MitraClip may potentially result in significant stenosis.[4] Detailed indications and relative contraindications have been previously published and is beyond the scope of this review.[4] Preprocedure imaging should also establish baseline ventricular function, exclude intracardiac thrombus, and determine the presence of baseline pericardial effusion. The imager should also

Table 1
Immediate preprocedural checklist to be performed after anesthesia and endotracheal tube placement, before initiation of procedural steps

	Immediate Preprocedural Checklist
1	Confirm MR severity, mechanism and origin. Become familiar with key TEE guidance views: bicommissural, long-axis, 3D en face, MPR, bicaval, AV short axis
2	Evaluate for pulmonary vein flow reversal
3	Measure MV gradient, and area using 3D planimetry
4	Rule out left atrial appendage thrombus
5	Evaluate for pericardial effusion
6	Evaluate interatrial septum for challenging anatomy

optimize and become familiar with key echocardiographic views to facilitate swift intraprocedural imaging. The key views include the bicaval, aortic valve short axis, bicommissural, long axis, and 3D views. An on-axis bicommissural view is crucial to understand the medial–lateral origin of the MR jet, and biplane imaging allows simultaneous visualization of a long axis view to understand anterior and posterior leaflet anatomy and MR mechanism (**Fig. 3**A, B). A 3D en face view provides visualization of overall mitral anatomy, and pathology such as prolapse or flail (**Fig. 3**C). Multiplanar reconstruction (MPR) is a technique to simultaneously visualize multiple 2D imaging planes based on and along with a 3D dataset. The MPR planes can be aligned to display all key mitral views, including the long axis, bicommissural, short axis and 3D en face (**Fig. 3**D, E). The use of this technique with and without color Doppler allows a determination of the MR mechanism and origin with precision. A limitation to note when using 3D imaging is that there is some loss of spatial and temporal resolution compared with 2D imaging, and so 3D images should be used in conjunction with standard 2D views.

Step 2: transseptal puncture

The TSP is a critical step because the location establishes the trajectory of the device for the rest of the procedure. An optimal puncture will facilitate maneuvering of the device within the left atrium (LA) to establish an ideal alignment and trajectory with the MV (**Fig. 4**), whereas a suboptimal TSP can create multiple challenges that need to be overcome during the course of the procedure. The standard TEE views during TSP guidance are the bicaval view for visualization of the superior–inferior axis, the short axis aortic valve view for the anterior–posterior axis, and the 4-chamber view for measurement of TSP height (**Fig. 5**).

During the first step of the procedure, the catheter starts in the SVC. The interventionalist then slowly withdraws the catheter inferiorly into the right atrium to approach the interatrial septum (IAS). The primary imaging view at this point is the bicaval view to find the tip of the catheter, indicated by tenting of the IAS (see **Fig. 5**, arrows). The ideal TSP location is within the mid to superior portion of the fossa ovalis. Once the superior–inferior position is satisfactory, one moves to the short axis aortic valve view for anterior–posterior positioning. This maneuver can be done by changing the primary image to a short axis of the aortic valve or with the use of biplane imaging or live MPR (see **Fig. 5**). A posterior puncture is preferred to optimize height above the MV and the trajectory

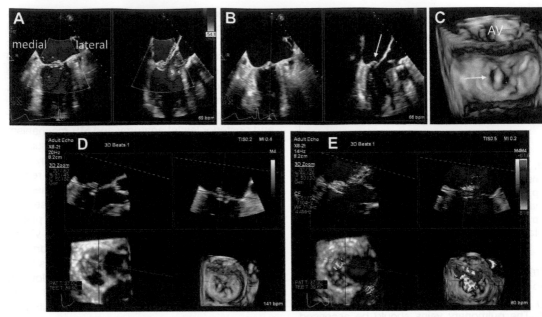

Fig. 3. Preprocedural evaluation of MR. (*A*) The MR origin is identified in the bicommissural view, which lays out the valve from medial to lateral. Biplane imaging is used to visualize the long axis view of the MR jet at this location. (*B*) Color Doppler is turned off to evaluate the underlying MV anatomy and determine the MR mechanism, in this case posterior leaflet prolapse and flail (*arrow*). (*C*) Three-dimensional en face view demonstrates P2 prolapse and flail (*arrow*). (*D*) Three-dimensional MPR shows all key views simultaneously, long axis (*upper left*), bicommissural (*upper right*), short axis (*lower left*) and 3D en face (*lower right*). (*E*) Three-dimensional MPR with color shows MR origin in all key views simultaneously (*E*).

in the LA. Last, the height is measured, as visualized at 0°, in the mid esophageal 4-chamber view (see **Fig. 5**B). The ideal TSP height is 4 to 5 cm above the target grasping zone of the MV.

Note that very medial pathology requires a high TSP to allow enough room for the clip delivery system (CDS) to bend back toward the septum without crossing into the left ventricle. Conversely,

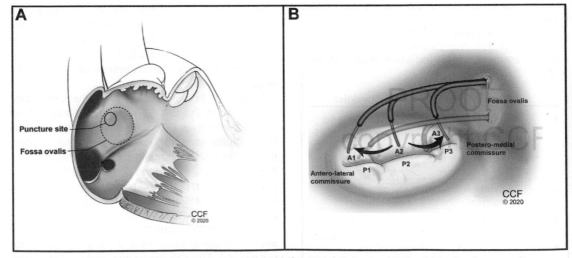

Fig. 4. Optimal TSP height showing trajectory toward the MV. (*A*) Optimal TSP within the fossa ovalis as seen from the right atrium. (*B*) Demonstration of TSP height for medial versus lateral pathology. If the TSP is too low (too close to the valve), there will not be room to adjust the device in the left atrium without crossing into the left ventricle. (Reprinted with permission, Cleveland Clinic Center for Medical Art & Photography ©2020. All Rights Reserved.)

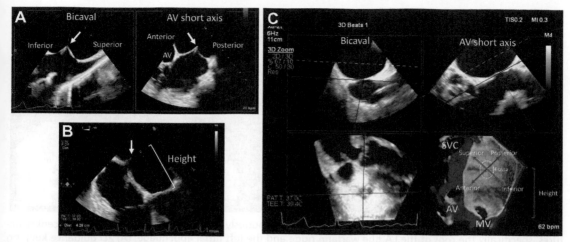

Fig. 5. Interatrial septal anatomy and guidance of the TSP. (*A*) The key views for guidance of the TSP include the bicaval view for superior–inferior axis (*left*) and the aortic valve short axis view for the anterior–posterior axis (*right*). The location of the needle is visualized by tenting of the septum (*arrows*). (*B*) The height is measured in the 4-chamber view from the tip of the mitral leaflets parallel to the septum until the level of the tenting. (*C*) Live MPR can be used to visualize all key views simultaneously. Movement along the superior–inferior and anterior–posterior axes in relationship to the MV height is demonstrated in the lower right image. Note that movement posteriorly, away from the AV, gains height above the MV. AV, aortic valve; SVC, superior vena cava.

the lateral pathology is more forgiving with regard to TSP height (see **Fig. 4**B).

Once the proposed TSP site is satisfactory, the needle is advanced across the IAS. In addition to visualizing the needle on the left atrial aspect of the IAS, other supportive findings of successful puncture include resolution of tenting and/or visualization of bubbles in the LA.

It is important that the TSP needle is continuously monitored to avoid inadvertent damage to adjacent structures such as the LA free wall and aortic root.

Other anatomic challenges to consider include a patent foramen ovale, atrial septal defect or aneurysm, or septal hypertrophy.[5] Crossing through a patent foramen ovale risks tearing the IAS and also may create a trajectory of the guide hugging

the anterior and superior wall of the LA. In the case of a septal aneurysm or mobile septum, applying pressure with the transseptal needle may bring it dangerously close to the LA free wall. In the presence of atrial septal hypertrophy, it is important to find the thin central portion of the fossa ovalis or use of a radiofrequency needle to facilitate puncture without exerting excessive force.[6]

After successful TSP, the guidewire is advanced into the left upper pulmonary vein or curled in the LA for stability. A 24F SGC with a dilator is then advanced to the septum (**Fig. 6**A).[4] It is important to monitor the tip of the guide crossing the septum, indicated by a double-density sign, as opposed to the dilator, which is cone shaped with multiple ridges This step can be performed with 2D imaging

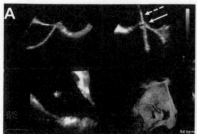
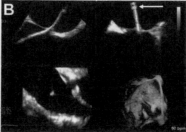
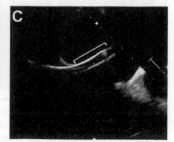

Fig. 6. Live MPR guidance of the SGC crossing the interatrial septum. (*A*) The guide tip is visualized on the right atrial side of the interatrial septum, indicated by the double density sign (*arrows*) along with tenting of the septum. The dilator is cone shaped with ridges (*dashed arrow*). (*B*) The guide tip has crossed into the LA with resolution of tenting. (*C*) The length of guide across the septum is measured.

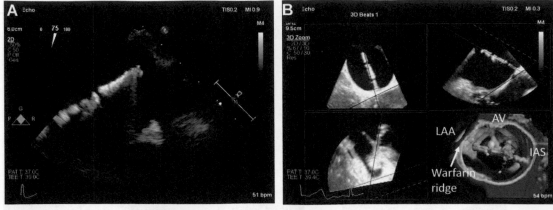

Fig. 7. Guiding the CDS within the LA. The clip must be continuously monitored to avoid injury to adjacent structures, specifically the roof of the LA, the warfarin ridge and the left atrial appendage. (*A*) 2D guidance keeping the tip of the clip in view to avoid injury to the LA free wall. (*B*) Live MPR guidance showing the CDS and key LA structures. AV, aortic valve; LAA, left atrial appendage.

from the bicaval view or with live MPR (see **Fig. 6**A) When the guide has crossed the septum, the tenting disappears, and the double-density will be visualized clearly within the LA (**Fig. 6**B). It is important to lay out the length of the guide from the tip to the septum and at minimum the catheter should be advanced approximately 2 to 3 cm into the LA. This positioning should be monitored consistently throughout the procedure to prevent inadvertent retraction into the right atrium (**Fig. 6**C).

Step 3: advance the clip delivery system into the left atrium

The CDS is then advanced out of the guide until straddling (as seen on fluoroscopy), at which point

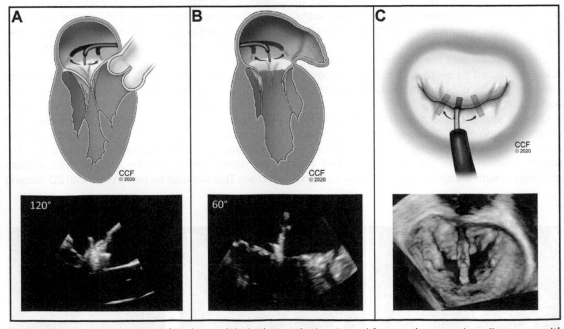

Fig. 8. Alignment of the CDS within the LA. (*A*) The long axis view is used for anterior-posterior adjustment, with anterior toward the AV and posterior away. (*B*) The bicommissural view is used for medial-lateral adjustment until the CDS is located above the target grasping zone. (*C*) The 3D *en face* view is used to adjust clip orientation with rotation of the clip clockwise or counterclockwise until perpendicular to leaflet coaptation. If the target is lateral, the clip typically needs clockwise rotation. Conversely, if the target is medial, the clip typically needs counterclockwise rotation. LA, left atrium. (Reprinted with permission, Cleveland Clinic Center for Medical Art & Photography ©2020. All Rights Reserved.)

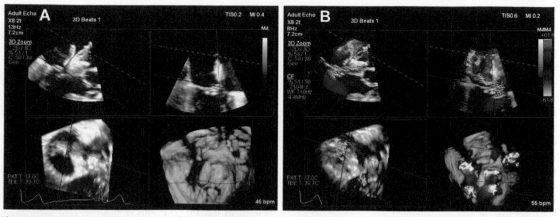

Fig. 9. Positioning and alignment of the clip in the LA using MPR. (*A*) Live MPR is used to simultaneously visualize all key views for alignment of the CDS in the LA: long axis view (*upper left*), bicommissural view (*upper right*), short axis view (*lower left*) and 3D *en face* lower right. The green plane is aligned with the clip arms in the short axis and 3D views to display the arms in the open position. (*B*) Once standard views are obtained and clip is aligned to target, color Doppler is added to confirm that the clip is aimed at the MR jet. LA, left atrium.

it can be steered down toward the MV. It is important to image the distal end of the CDS as it exits the SGC into the LA to avoid contact with the roof of the LA. Once the CDS is advanced sufficiently out of the guide, the clip is continuously tracked as it is steered down toward the MV. During this maneuver, the clip, LA appendage, and the warfarin ridge need to be visualized to ensure the clip does not catch the warfarin ridge or the left atrial appendage (**Fig. 7**A). Real-time 3D

echocardiography can be useful to visualize the aforementioned structures in a single view (**Fig. 7**B).

Step 4: adjust the clip position and orientation
Once the CDS is advanced toward the MV, the next step is to position and orient the clip in the LA (**Fig. 8**). Manipulation within the left ventricle (LV) is minimized to prevent injury to the subvalvular apparatus. The key views for position the clip in

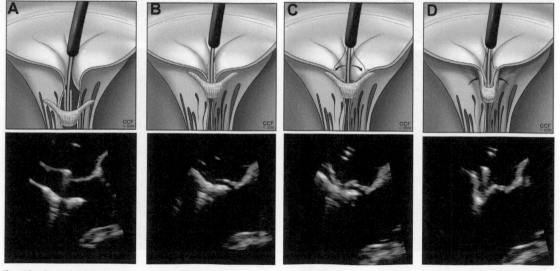

Fig. 10. Grasping sequence. (*A*) The clip is advanced into the LV. (*B*) The clip is slowly withdrawn back toward the LA until anterior and posterior leaflets are resting above clip arms. (*C*) The grippers are lowered to trap the leaflets between the grippers and the clip arms. (*D*) The clip arms are closed to appose the anterior and posterior leaflets. LA, left atrium; LV, left ventricle. (Reprinted with permission, Cleveland Clinic Center for Medical Art & Photography ©2020. All Rights Reserved.)

the LA include the long axis view for anterior–posterior position (see **Fig. 8**A) and the bicommissural view for medial–lateral position (see **Fig. 8**B). Last, the clip orientation is visualized using a 3D en face view (see **Fig. 8**C) and is rotated clockwise or counterclockwise until it is perpendicular to leaflet coaptation. It is important to note that, if the clip is placed centrally, along A2 to P2, the clip orientation will be straight up and down; however, if the clip is placed medially, along A3 to P3, the clip typically requires counterclockwise rotation to remain perpendicular to the coaptation zone. Conversely, clockwise rotation is necessary when targeting lateral pathology, such as A1 to P1 (see **Fig. 8**C)

Biplane imaging allows simultaneously visualization of the long axis and bicommissural views. Alternatively, live 3D MPR is a powerful tool because a single 3D dataset can be used to simultaneously visualize all key views, including the long axis, bicommissural, and short axis views, along with the 3D en face view (**Fig. 9**A). Before advancing into the ventricle, assessment using color Doppler should be used to confirm the clip position relative to MR origin (**Fig. 9**B).

Step 5: advancing the clip into the left ventricle and leaflet capture

With the clips arms and both mitral leaflets visualized, the clip is advanced across the MV into the LV. At this stage, it is critical to provide high-quality long axis images of the MV showing anterior and posteriorly leaflets as well as the anterior and posterior clip arms. This process can be done using single plane imaging, biplane imaging, or live MPR. Once in the LV, the clip is then slowly withdrawn back toward the LA until both leaflets are resting just above the clip arms in systole and diastole. The grippers are then lowered and one should pay close attention to the amount of anterior and posterior leaflets inserted in between the clip arms and grippers. The clip arms are then closed

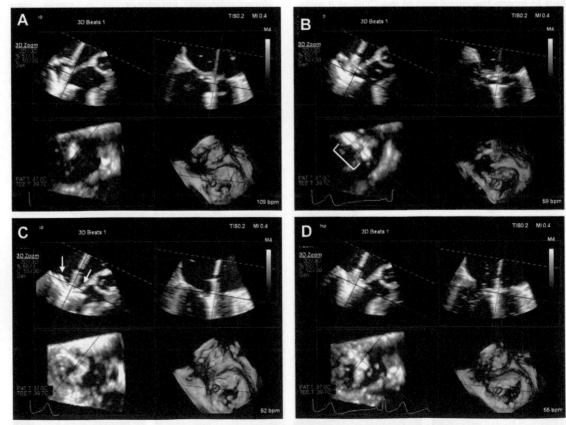

Fig. 11. Live MPR for guidance of leaflet grasping. (*A*) The green plane is aligned with the clip to show the long axis grasping view with clear visualization of both clip arms as well as anterior and posterior leaflets. (*B*) The clip is withdrawn back toward the LA until both mitral leaflets are resting on top of open clip arms. Note that within the blue plane, one can clearly visualize that the green grasping plane is aligned with the open clip arms (bracket) confirming on axis grasping views. (*C*) Grippers are lowered with leaflets inserted in between clip arms and grippers (*arrows*). (*D*) Clip is closed. Both anterior and posteriorly leaflets are immobilized.

(**Fig. 10**). Historically, these steps are guided using single or biplane imaging. Recently, live MPR has shown to be a powerful tool to simultaneously monitor all aspects of clip position and orientation during this crucial stage of the procedure (**Fig. 11**).[7]

If, during the grasping sequence, it becomes difficult to image the clip, it is important to recognize that the clip position or orientation may have changed as it crossed the valve. The bicommissural view and 3D en face views may be helpful to evaluate for any changes in device location. When using live MPR, as opposed to single plane or biplane imaging, the clip position and orientation are monitored continuously, so that if changes occur, they are recognized immediately and corrected.

If leaflet capture is challenging, there are several maneuvers that can be helpful. If there is a large flail gap in systole, prolongation of diastole with adenosine may be beneficial to bringing the leaflets closer together for grasping.[8] Conversely, if the problem is severe restriction of the leaflets in

diastole, then rapid pacing to hold the leaflets closer together in the systolic phase may be helpful.[9] Breath-holding, with or without a Valsalva maneuver, may also be used to decrease the translational motion of the heart, which may in turn improve the ease of grasping.

Step 6: assessment of leaflet capture and residual mitral regurgitation

Once the leaflets are grasped, the next step is to determine if the device should be released (left in place) or repositioned. This decision is based on whether there is appropriate leaflet capture and adequate reduction in MR, while avoiding the development of mitral stenosis.

Leaflet grasp should be carefully assessed with multiple 2D and 3D views. The key 2D views are the long axis and 4-chamber views, demonstrating immobilization of both leaflets within the device (**Fig. 12**A, B). Another technique is to find the clip in the bicommissural view and then biplane through the device to show the long axis view in

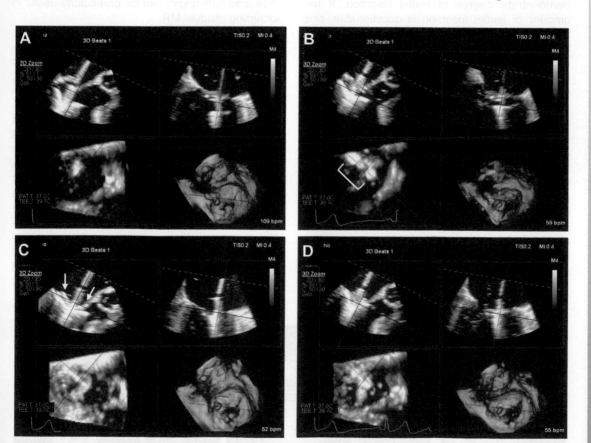

Fig. 12. Assessment of leaflet grasp. Grasp of anterior and posterior leaflets should be confirmed by demonstrating immobilization of leaflets within the device in multiple views, including (*A*) 0°, (*B*) long axis, (*C*) bicommissural view with biplane imaging, and (*D*) live MPR. Note that within the blue plane in panel B, one can clearly visualize that the green grasping plane is aligned with the open clip arms (bracket) confirming on axis grasping views. In panel C, capture and immobilization of the leaflets are demonstrated after lowering of the grippers (*arrows*).

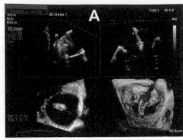
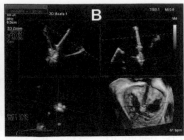
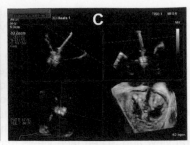

Fig. 13. Measurement of leaflet length to determine leaflet insertion. (*A*) The length of the posterior leaflet was measured before grasping, 1.5 cm. The remaining leaflet outside of the device was measured after grasping, 1.1 cm (*B*). The difference between leaflet length pre and post grasp was used to estimate the amount of leaflet inserted in the device. In this case, inadequate leaflet insertion was noted, only 4 mm. (*C*) Leaflet grasp was optimized and the posterior leaflet was remeasured, 0.8 cm, for over 0.6 cm leaflet insertion within the device.

the orthogonal plane (**Fig. 12**C). Again, live MPR is a particularly useful too at this juncture, given its ability to simultaneously display all the key views (**Fig. 12**D). Of note, a 3D en face view is helpful to show clip position and creation of a double orifice valve; however, this view alone cannot demonstrate degree of leaflet insertion. If the amount of leaflet insertion is questionable, one technique is to measure the baseline leaflet length before grasping and then compare it with the residual leaflet length outside of the clip after grasping (**Fig. 13**). Examples of poor leaflet capture are provided in **Fig. 14**. Single leaflet detachment can occur in between 1% and 5% of cases,[10,11] and so it is critical to confirm appropriate leaflet grasp before device deployment.

Residual MR is assessed using conventional methods,[12] including evaluation of proximal flow convergence and pulmonary venous flow pattern. A recent study has also demonstrated the utility of 3D vena contracta in assessing residual MR after MitraClip.[13] Invasive hemodynamics, including change in LA pressure after MitraClip placement, is also an important metric to consider.[14]

Significant residual MR (>2+) should be evaluated carefully to determine the mechanism and etiology, as well as exact location, and specifically whether the origin is medial or lateral to the device. Either a bicommissural view with biplane imaging or live MPR are the best imaging tools to answer these questions (**Fig. 15**). A 3D view from the ventricle to visualize the proximal isovelocity surface area (MR origin) can be particularly useful in localizing residual MR.

If the residual MR is felt to be secondary to poor leaflet capture or incorrect placement, then the clip should be removed and repositioned. If clip position and leaflet capture are felt to be adequate, but additional pathology remains, then the anatomy should be evaluated to determine the suitability for additional clip placement. One must consider 2 factors in this situation: is the residual pathology graspable and is the residual MV orifice sufficient to accommodate an additional device without development of mitral stenosis. The target mitral gradient is less than 5 mm Hg because a mean mitral gradient of more than 5 mm Hg after the MitraClip is associated with adverse long-term outcomes.[15] If the gradient is more than 5 mm Hg, one may try to slow the heart rate and reassess. In addition, 3D planimetry can be used to directly measure residual MVA. Because the 2

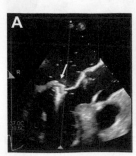
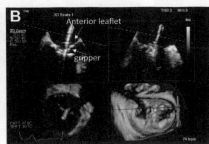
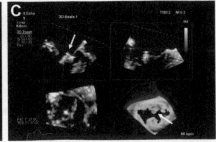

Fig. 14. Examples of poor leaflet insertion. Only tip of posterior leaflet captured (*A, arrow*). Anterior leaflet inserted above, not below gripper (*B*). Single leaflet detachment with clip only attached to anterior and not posterior leaflet (*C, arrows*).

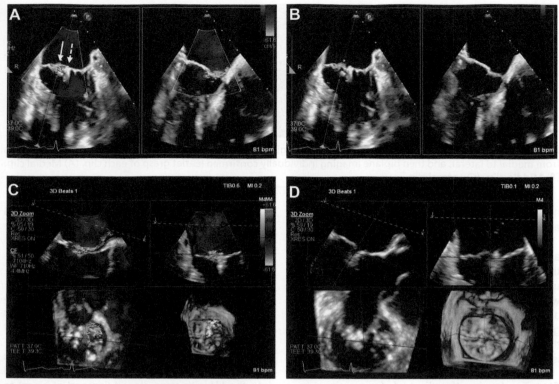

Fig. 15. Localization of residual MR and simulation of grasping view. (*A*) The bicommissural view demonstrates residual MR (*arrow*) medial to the device (*dashed arrow*). Biplane imaging shows the MR in long axis. (*B*) When color Doppler is turned off, MV anatomy can be assessed to understand mechanism of MR and suitability of anatomy for additional device. (*C*) Live MPR can be used to assess residual MR by aligning the green and red planes through the MR origin. (*D*) Color Doppler is then turned off to assess underlying leaflet anatomy at the MR origin to assess graspability at that location. Note that Live MPR shows a precise grasping view (green plane) compared with the biplane long axis view that appears off axis without clear LVOT and AV in view. AV, aortic valve; LVOT, left ventricular outflow tract.

orifices may lie in different planes, each mitral orifice should be measured independently using 3D MPR, and then the 2 areas can be added for total residual MVA (**Fig. 16**). To answer the question of graspability of the residual pathology, one can simulate a potential grasping view by first localizing the residual MR with color Doppler, using either biplane imaging from the bicommissural view or live MPR, and then turning color off to understand the underlying leaflet anatomy (see **Fig. 15**). This assessment should be performed before releasing the clip. If an additional clip is

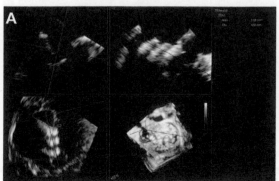
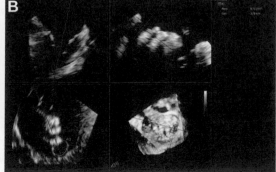

Fig. 16. Assessment of residual MVA by 3D planimetry. The (*A*) lateral and (*B*) medial orifices should be measured individually to calculate residual MVA.

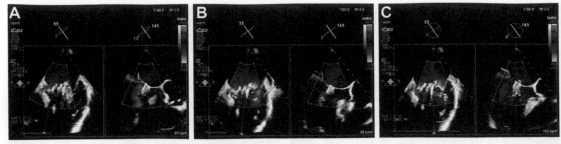

Fig. 17. Assessment of individual clips using biplane imaging. The bicommissural view was used to visualize 3 clips from medial to lateral, and then biplane imaging individually confirmed leaflet grasp of each clip. (*A*) Medial clip. (*B*) Middle clip. (*C*) Lateral clip.

not possible, then one may wish to consider adjusting the current clip for a better result.

In summary, clip placement is felt to be adequate for release if (1) good leaflet grasp at the target pathology (2) Mitral gradient and residual MVA is adequate (post clip MVA of >1.5 cm^2 with a mean transmitral gradient of <5 mm Hg), and (3) a significant decrease in MR by at least 1 grade to no more than moderate (2+) MR,[16] or if there is significant residual MR, an additional clip is anatomically feasible.

Step 7: releasing the clip and closing views

After the clip is released, the MV should be reassessed because residual MR and the mitral gradient may change after tension from the CDS is removed. The LV ejection fraction may also decrease after clip deployment given the increased afterload as a result of decreased regurgitant flow into the LA. For this reason, with each clip, both before and after, the degree of residual MR, pulmonary venous Doppler and LV function should be reassessed.

Once satisfied with the mitral result, the CDS and SGC are withdrawn across the IAS under TEE guidance.

SPECIAL CONSIDERATIONS
Placement of Additional Clips

Imaging guidance for placement of additional clips can be technically challenging because artifact from the first clip can make visualization of adjacent leaflets challenging. The additional clip is positioned and oriented in the LA, then advanced into the LV with arms closed (instead of open) to avoid disrupting the prior clip. It is important to ensure that the correct clip is being visualized during grasping and assessment of leaflet capture, because it is easy to confuse 2 adjacent clips, especially once closed. Both biplane (**Fig. 17**) and 3D MPR (**Fig. 18**) imaging are essential to allow detailed assessment of each individual clip. The sole use of single plane 2D imaging increases the possibility of evaluating the incorrect clip and missing inadequate leaflet capture.

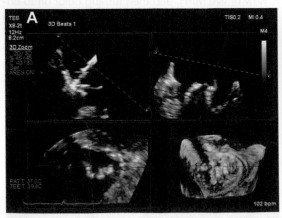
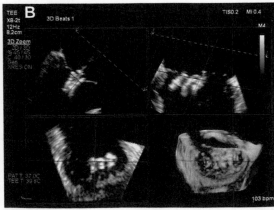

Fig. 18. Live MPR for placement of additional clips. (*A*) Live MPR was used for grasping during placement of a third MitraClip device laterally. The grasping plane (*upper left*) shows insertion of anterior and posterior leaflets within the arms and grippers. (*B*) Leaflet grasp was confirmed using Live MPR. All 3 devices are clearly seen on bicommissural (*upper right*) and short axis (*lower left*) views, with the long axis green plane (*upper left*) aligned to confirm grasp of anterior and posterior leaflets.

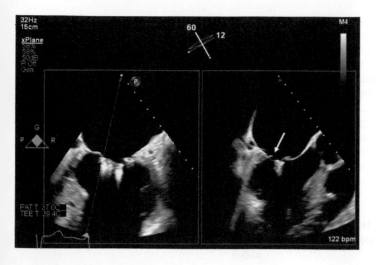

Fig. 19. Leaflet tear. Biplane imaging through the medial clip shows the grasp of this clip, which in this case demonstrates a leaflet tear (*arrow*), as indicated by the very short residual posterior leaflet with flail.

Immediate Complications

The MitraClip procedure is overall a very safe procedure; however, there are several complications of which one must be aware. There is a risk of LA injury during TSP and with the movement of the equipment in the LA. For this reason, if hypotension occurs, one should quickly evaluate for the development of pericardial effusion and tamponade. When the clip is manipulated in the LV, it is possible for injury to the subvalvular apparatus to occur, which could lead to a chordal tear. This complication should be considered if MR changes in character or severity during the procedure. Another potential etiology of worsening MR is leaflet injury, such as leaflet tear, that can occur during grasping (**Fig. 19**). If MR worsens after clip release, then it is also important to consider the possibility of single leaflet detachment, which can occur secondary to either a leaflet tear or poor leaflet insertion (see **Fig. 14**C).

At the completion of the procedure, the residual iatrogenic atrial septal defect should be evaluated for size and direction of shunt flow. A previous study of a small series of patients showed an association of large residual defect (>10 mm) with increased morbidity and mortality, so atrial septal defect closure may be considered in these patients.[17] Significant right-to-left shunting with hypoxia is another indication for closure.

DISCLOSURE

The authors have nothing to disclose.

REFERENCES

1. Stone GW, Lindenfeld J, Abraham WT, et al. Transcatheter mitral-valve repair in patients with heart failure. N Engl J Med 2018;379:2307–18.

2. Ramchand J, Harb SC, Krishnaswamy A, et al. Echocardiographic guidance of transcatheter mitral valve edge-to-edge repair. Struct Heart 2020;4: 397–412.

3. Ho SY. Anatomy of the mitral valve. Heart 2002; 88(Suppl 4):iv5–10.

4. Wunderlich NC, Siegel RJ. Peri-interventional echo assessment for the MitraClip procedure. Eur Heart J Cardiovasc Imaging 2013;14:935–49.

5. Ramchand J, Harb SC, Miyasaka R, et al. Imaging for percutaneous left atrial appendage closure: a contemporary review. Struct Heart 2019;3:364–82.

6. Tokuda M, Yamashita S, Matsuo S, et al. Radiofrequency needle for transseptal puncture is associated with lower incidence of thromboembolism during catheter ablation of atrial fibrillation: propensity score-matched analysis. Heart Vessels 2018; 33:1238–44.

7. Harb SC, Krishnaswamy A, Kapadia SR, et al. The added value of 3D real-time multiplanar reconstruction for intraprocedural guidance of challenging MitraClip cases. JACC Cardiovasc Imaging 2020;13: 1809–14.

8. Borgia F, Di Mario C, Franzen O. Adenosine-induced asystole to facilitate MitraClip placement in a patient with adverse mitral valve morphology. Heart 2011; 97:864.

9. Hahn RT. Transcathether valve replacement and valve repair: review of procedures and intraprocedural echocardiographic imaging. Circ Res 2016; 119:341–56.

10. Maisano F, Franzen O, Baldus S, et al. Percutaneous mitral valve interventions in the real world: early and 1-year results from the ACCESS-EU, a prospective, multicenter, nonrandomized post-approval study of the MitraClip therapy in Europe. J Am Coll Cardiol 2013;62:1052–61.

11. Sorajja P, Mack M, Vemulapalli S, et al. Initial experience with commercial transcatheter mitral valve repair in the United States. J Am Coll Cardiol 2016;67:1129–40.

12. Zoghbi WA, Adams D, Bonow RO, et al. Recommendations for noninvasive evaluation of native valvular regurgitation: a report from the American Society of Echocardiography Developed in Collaboration with the Society for Cardiovascular Magnetic Resonance. J Am Soc Echocardiogr 2017;30:303–71.

13. Avenatti E, Mackensen GB, El-Tallawi KC, et al. Diagnostic Value of 3-dimensional vena contracta area for the quantification of residual mitral regurgitation after MitraClip procedure. JACC Cardiovasc Interv 2019;12:582–91.

14. Siegel RJ, Biner S, Rafique AM, et al. The acute hemodynamic effects of MitraClip therapy. J Am Coll Cardiol 2011;57:1658–65.

15. Neuss M, Schau T, Isotani A, et al. Elevated Mitral Valve Pressure Gradient after MitraClip implantation deteriorates long-term outcome in patients with severe mitral regurgitation and severe heart failure. JACC Cardiovasc Interv 2017;10:931–9.

16. Stone GW, Adams DH, Abraham WT, et al. Clinical trial design principles and endpoint definitions for transcatheter mitral valve repair and replacement: part 2: endpoint definitions: a consensus document from the mitral valve academic research consortium. J Am Coll Cardiol 2015;66:308–21.

17. Schueler R, Ozturk C, Wedekind JA, et al. Persistence of iatrogenic atrial septal defect after interventional mitral valve repair with the MitraClip system: a note of caution. JACC Cardiovasc Interv 2015;8:450–9.

Looking into the Mechanistic Link Between Mitral Regurgitation and Atrial Fibrillation

Yukio Abe, MD, PhD[a],*, Yosuke Takahashi, MD, PhD[b],
Toshihiko Shibata, MD, PhD[b]

KEYWORDS

- Atrial fibrillation • Atrial functional mitral regurgitation • Echocardiography • Heart failure
- Valvular heart disease

KEY POINTS

- Atrial functional mitral regurgitation can occur in patients with atrial fibrillation despite a preserved left ventricular systolic function.
- Atrial functional mitral regurgitation is an important cause of heart failure and a considerable therapeutic target in patients with heart failure with atrial fibrillation.
- Mitral annular dilatation owing to atrial fibrillation-induced left atrial dilatation is primarily necessary for the generation of atrial functional mitral regurgitation.
- Hamstringing of the posterior mitral leaflet also relates to the generation of atrial functional mitral regurgitation.
- Further mitral annular dilatation owing to progressive dilatations of the left atrium and left ventricle, with mitral regurgitation-induced volume overload, worsens atrial functional mitral regurgitation.

INTRODUCTION

Primary mitral regurgitation (MR), when significant, can lead to the occurrence of atrial fibrillation (AF) owing to the left atrial (LA) volume/pressure overload. Therefore, atrial fibrillation can be viewed as evidence of the pathologic significance of primary MR, and the presence of concomitant severe primary MR and new-onset atrial fibrillation is considered a sign of a surgical indication for MR.[1,2] Conversely, MR can also occur as a consequence of LA dilatation in patients with atrial fibrillation. This type of secondary MR and its mechanistic link with atrial fibrillation are the topic of discussion in the present review article.

DEFINITION OF ATRIAL FUNCTIONAL MITRAL REGURGITATION

Secondary MR (ie, functional MR) was originally identified as resulting from mitral leaflet tethering–tenting owing to left ventricular (LV) systolic dysfunction and remodeling in patients with ischemic heart disease or dilated cardiomyopathy.[3–5] One long-held belief is that atrial fibrillation, on its own, sometimes causes significant functional tricuspid regurgitation (TR), but does not usually cause significant functional MR.[6,7] By contrast, several studies have recently shown that functional MR can occur in patients with atrial fibrillation and an enlarged LA, despite a lack of

[a] Department of Cardiology, Osaka City General Hospital, 2-13-22 Miyakojima-hondori, Miyakojima-ku, Osaka 534-0021, Japan; [b] Department of Cardiovascular Surgery, Osaka City University, 1-4-3 Asahimachi, Abeno-ku, Osaka 545-8585, Japan
* Corresponding author.
E-mail address: abeyukio@aol.com

Cardiol Clin 39 (2021) 281–288
https://doi.org/10.1016/j.ccl.2021.01.010

LV systolic dysfunction.[8–22] This occurrence can be termed atrial functional MR (AFMR) and has received much attention as an important cause of heart failure. It is also a considerable therapeutic target in patients with heart failure with persistent atrial fibrillation and preserved LV ejection fraction (LVEF). The traditional functional MR occurring in patients with LV dilatation and/or systolic dysfunction has sometimes been termed ventricular functional MR (VFMR) to distinguish it from AFMR.[15,21]

AFMR can be defined as MR with:

- LA dilatation, mainly seen in patients with atrial fibrillation;
- No significant degenerative change in the mitral valve complex; and
- No significant LV systolic dysfunction or dilatation.

However, no cut-off values for LVEF and LV size have yet been established to rule in/out AFMR. Most previous studies that have examined AFMR have used 50% as the cut-off value for LVEF. Some studies have also used the cut-off value of the LV diastolic diameter or volume using various references that established the normal values to study pure AFMR.[10,11,13] In real-world clinical settings, however, patients with AFMR can have a dilated LV owing to the volume overload resulting from chronic MR. Patients with AFMR can also have a decreased LVEF in the advanced stage. Therefore, patients with mild LV dilatation or mild LV systolic dysfunction should also be recognized as having AFMR if they have functional MR that originates from LA dilatation rather than from LV dilatation or systolic dysfunction.[20,21]

Patients with sinus rhythm can also have AFMR owing to LA dilatation resulting from LV diastolic dysfunction rather than from atrial fibrillation, whereas significant AFMR is thought to be less prevalent in patients with sinus rhythm than in patients with atrial fibrillation. Tamargo and colleagues[23] studied 280 patients with heart failure with a preserved LVEF and showed that patients with mild to moderate functional MR had a higher prevalence of atrial fibrillation than did patients with no to trivial functional MR (38% vs 13%; P<.0001). Surprisingly, the remaining 62% of the patients with heart failure with a preserved LVEF and mild to moderate functional MR had a sinus rhythm. The true distribution of the sinus rhythm and atrial fibrillation in patients with AFMR remains unknown because patients with more than moderate MR were excluded from the study.

PREVALENCE AND PROGNOSIS OF PATIENTS WITH ATRIAL FUNCTIONAL MITRAL REGURGITATION

We found that the prevalence of significant AFMR was 8.1% in patients with atrial fibrillation who underwent transthoracic echocardiography but were without other underlying heart diseases or reduced LVEF, whereas the prevalence was 28% for patients with longstanding persistent atrial fibrillation (duration >10 years) (**Fig. 1**).[14] This difference was greater than expected. The event-free rate for cardiac death or hospitalization for worsening heart failure was not high (53%), even at a follow-up of only 24 months, in patients with significant AFMR (**Fig. 2**A). Patients with significant AFMR in conjunction with secondary TR had the poorest prognosis, with an event-free rate of 27% at 24 months (**Fig. 2**B).

TR owing to right atrial dilatation and tricuspid annular dilatation is also referred to as atrial functional TR (AFTR). The combination of AFMR and AFTR, which had the poorest prognosis, should therefore receive greater therapeutic attention. Some other studies have reported that patients with persistent atrial fibrillation who were hospitalized owing to heart failure with preserved EF had significant AFMR more frequently (37%–44%), even at discharge after medical therapies, and their AFMR was associated with readmission owing to heart failure during the postdischarge follow-up.[15,16] Dziadzko and colleagues,[20] in a study of 727 residents living in a community,

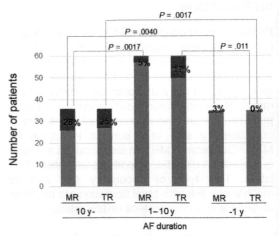

Fig. 1. Prevalence of significant (ie, moderate or greater) MR or TR versus duration of AF. *Blue*, not significant; *orange*, significant. (*From* Abe Y, Akamatsu K, Ito K, et al. Prevalence and prognostic significance of functional mitral and tricuspid regurgitation despite preserved left ventricular ejection fraction in atrial fibrillation patients. Circ J. 2018;82:1451–8; with permission.)

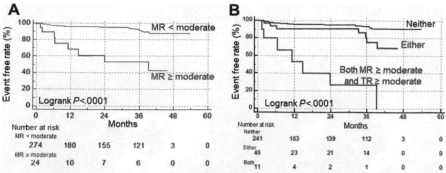

Fig. 2. Kaplan–Meier event-free rates of cardiac death, hospitalization owing to worsening heart failure (*A*) by the status of significant (ie, moderate or greater) mitral regurgitation (MR); and (*B*) by the status of significant MR or TR. (*From* Abe Y, Akamatsu K, Ito K, et al. Prevalence and prognostic significance of functional mitral and tricuspid regurgitation despite preserved left ventricular ejection fraction in atrial fibrillation patients. Circ J. 2018;82:1451–8; with permission.)

reported that 32%, 38%, and 27% of the residents with a first diagnosis of isolated moderate or severe MR (determined by clinically indicated echocardiography) had organic MR, VFMR, and AFMR, respectively. The study also revealed a significantly increased prevalence of AFMR with patient age, and the AFMR was related to mortality or the incidence of heart failure. Kim and colleagues[24] recently reported better outcomes for medically treated patients with AFMR than with VFMR with LV dysfunction, but worse outcomes than patients with primary MR. Consequently, the appropriate diagnosis and treatment of AFMR will become more important in preventing cardiac death and heart failure in patients with atrial fibrillation in our aging societies.

ETIOLOGY OF ATRIAL FUNCTIONAL MITRAL REGURGITATION

The etiology of AFMR is the most important issue covered in this review article. Several recent studies have shown that LA dilatation and the subsequent mitral annular (MA) dilatation are both main etiologies of AFMR.[8–14,17–22] The fact that MA dilatation is not mainly induced by LV dilatation but by LA dilatation is not fully unknown.[22,25] Some may wonder why the LV connected with MA has less impact on MA than is observed with the LA. In fact, however, the MA that is defined as the edge at the root of the mitral leaflet is usually positioned at the junction of the LV and LA or at the LA wall, out of touch with the LV. By contrast, no MA is positioned at the LV wall out of touch with the LA. The phenomenon whereby the MA is positioned away from the LV edge is referred to as MA disjunction.[26–28] MA disjunction is not seen in all patients and is not homogenous, even in the same patient. The MA

dilatation owing to the LA dilation reduces the coaptation of the leaflets and is likely to generate MR with a central jet, corresponding to Carpentier type I MR (**Fig. 3**). The cut-off value for the MA dimension index for generating significant AFMR (moderate or more degrees) is 21 to 22 cm^2/m^2, as measured in the long axis view with transthoracic echocardiography.[22]

Other factors have also been suggested as etiologies of AFMR.[11–13,17,18,22] These factors include the disruption of the MA saddle shape,[11,17,18] a decrease in MA contractility,[11,18] inadequate compensation for the MA dilatation resulting from the lack of leaflet remodeling,[13,17] and tethering of the posterior mitral leaflet (PML).[11,12,22] However, the main determinants and the relationships among the various etiologies have not been fully elucidated.

Insufficient leaflet remodeling cannot compensate for the MA dilatation and can cause the generation and worsening of MR. An experimental histopathologic study and a clinical study have both confirmed that mitral leaflets expand to occlude systolic MA in patients with VFMR.[29,30] This phenomenon represents leaflet remodeling, and patients with significant VFMR have a smaller mitral leaflet closure to leaflet area ratio, which represents insufficient leaflet remodeling. The same findings have also been reported in 3-dimensional transesophageal echocardiography studies as an important etiology of AFMR without LV dysfunction.[13,17]

Our previous study using 3-dimensional transesophageal echocardiography showed that the anterior mitral leaflet (AML) was flattened along the MA plane and that the PML was bent toward the LV cavity at midsystole in patients with significant AFMR.[16] The LA dilates posteriorly, and the posterior MA is displaced backward to the LA

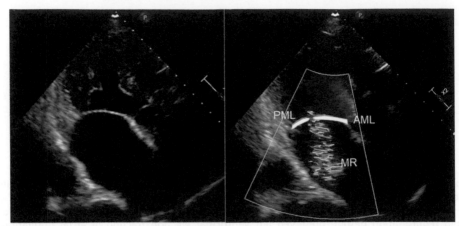

Fig. 3. Atrial functional mitral regurgitation with a flattened anterior mitral leaflet, flattened PML, and central mitral regurgitant (MR) jet (Carpentier I). AML, anterior mitral leaflet.

side from the crest of the posterior LV. This backward LA enlargement causes an inner bending of the basal posterior LV. The posterior displacement of the MA is emphasized at systole by the paradoxic posterior movement of the basal LV.[19] The tip of the PML then becomes tethered to the posterior LV by the papillary muscles and the chordae tendineae. This PML tethering that originates from LA dilatation is referred to as atriogenic leaflet tethering.[19] The result of this atriogenic leaflet tethering is a curving of the PML, which restricts its movement. This functional restriction of the PML was originally seen in patients with giant LA owing to rheumatic mitral valve disease and has traditionally been referred to as the hamstringing of the posterior cusp.[31] The PML hamstringing seen in the current patients with AFMR can be recognized as being more purely functional than that seen in patients with rheumatic mitral valve disease (**Fig. 4**).[12,21] Atriogenic leaflet tethering of the PML, complicated with MA dilatation, further decreases the leaflet coaptation, thereby deteriorating the MR. AFMR with PML hamstringing is classified as a combination of Carpentier type I for AML and type IIIb for PML and is likely to have an eccentric jet directed toward the posterior LA wall (see **Fig. 4**). The AML with a coaptation gap from the tethered PML in patients with AFMR with an eccentric jet can be considered to have a pseudoprolapse or override.

AFMR is defined as secondary MR with LA and MA dilatation and can be classified into 2 types: one has the flattened AML, a flattened PML, and a central jet, and the other has the flattened AML with pseudoprolapse, a tethered PML with the hamstringing phenomenon, and an eccentric jet (**Fig. 5**). The factors that divide these 2 types of AFMR remain unknown. Another recent article of

ours that included 159 consecutive patients with atrial fibrillation and preserved LVEF demonstrated that a total of 7 of 13 patients (54%) with significant AFMR had PML hamstringing, and 4 of the 7 patients with both significant MR and PML hamstringing had eccentric MR jets.[22] The findings in this article also suggested the following important information: (1) the systolic LV size, as well as the LA size, were the independent determinants of MR grading; (2) the MA size and the presence of the PML hamstringing were both the independent determinants of MR grading among the parameters of systolic mitral morphology; (3) the LA size was the strongest determinant of the MA size, but the LV size was also an independent determinant of the MA size; and (4) the LA size was associated with the hamstringing phenomenon of PML, whereas the LV systolic dimension index was not. These results have led us to now believe that both the MA dilatation and the PML hamstringing can occur owing to atrial fibrillation-induced LA dilatation and generate MR. Subsequently, additional LA and LV dilatations, which may be induced by volume overload owing to the MR, can lead to further dilatation of the MA and worsening of the MR (**Fig. 6**).[22]

TREATMENTS FOR PATIENTS WITH ATRIAL FUNCTIONAL MITRAL REGURGITATION

Recently published guidelines have not addressed the treatment of AFMR.[1,2] However, the Japanese guidelines for the treatments for valvular heart disease have been the first to address AFMR.[32] The new Japanese guidelines indicate that:

- Symptomatic patients with AFMR should first receive standard medical therapy for heart

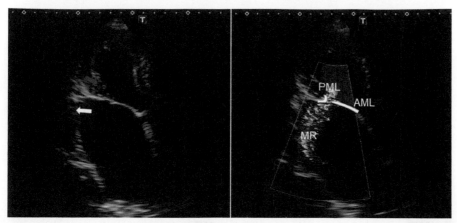

Fig. 4. Atrial functional mitral regurgitation (MR) with a flattened AML with pseudoprolapse, a tethered PML with the hamstringing phenomenon, and an eccentric MR jet (Carpentier I for AML and IIIb for PML). The left atrium (LA) dilates posteriorly (*white arrow*), and the posterior mitral annulus is displaced backward to the LA side from the crest of the posterior LV. This backward LA enlargement causes inner bending of the basal posterior left ventricle (*red arrow*).

failure, including diuretics (Class I but evidence level C);

- Atrial fibrillation catheter ablation is reasonable for symptomatic patients with persistent atrial fibrillation and severe AFMR, if successful ablation and maintenance of sinus rhythm can be expected from the duration of atrial fibrillation and the LA size (class IIa but evidence level C); and
- Mitral valve surgery is reasonable for patients with severe AFMR who are consistently symptomatic, despite standard medical therapy for heart failure (class IIa but evidence level C), and can also be applied to patients with chronic moderate AFMR if the MR is severe

upon worsening of the heart failure or during exercise stress tests.

Appropriate interventions for AFMR and AFTR may differ depending on the degree of atrial remodeling. However, an appropriate cut-off value for atrial size or some other parameter for selecting catheter ablation or surgery remains undetermined. The recommendation regarding atrial fibrillation catheter ablation is based on an article showing that maintaining a sinus rhythm with catheter ablation of the pulmonary veins can decrease the MR burden and decrease the LA volume and MA size in patients with both atrial fibrillation and AFMR.[9] The recommendation regarding mitral

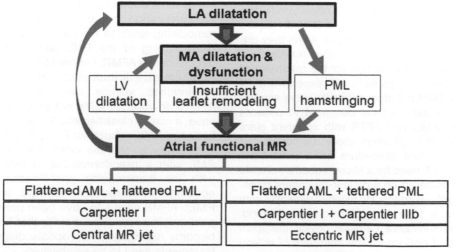

Fig. 5. Mechanisms and 2 types of atrial functional mitral regurgitation (MR).

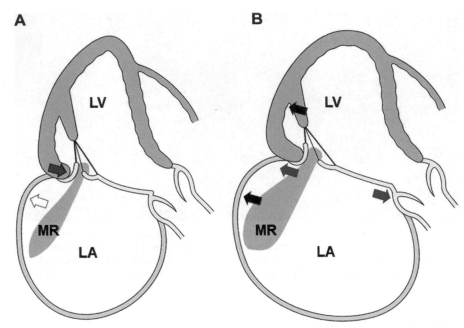

Fig. 6. Genesis and worsening of atrial functional mitral regurgitation (AFMR). (*A*) The left atrial (LA) posterior wall extends behind the posterior mitral annulus (MA) wlth LA dilatation (*white arrow*). The backward LA enlargement leads to an inward bending of the basal posterior left ventricle (LV) (*red arrow*). The posterior mitral annulus is displaced backward, whereas the tip of the PML is tethered toward the posterior LV. As a result, the PML curves and loses its functional mobility and coaptation with the AML (hamstringing). The result is generation of MR. This PML tethering is observed in a proportion, but not all, of the patients with AFMR and is likely to cause an eccentric jet directed toward the posterior LA wall. (*B*) Secondary LA and LV dilatations (*black arrows*), which may be induced by the MR, lead to further MA dilatation (*green arrows*) and worsening of the MR. (*From* Akamatsu K, Abe Y, Matsumura Y, et al. Etiology of atrial functional mitral regurgitation: insights from transthoracic echocardiography in 159 consecutive patients with atrial fibrillation and preserved left ventricular ejection fraction. Cardiology 2020;145:511–21; with permission.)

valve surgery is based on articles suggesting that surgical mitral valve repair may be useful in addressing AFMR and the coexisting heart failure.[10,33,34]

AFMR is likely to accompany secondary AFTR owing to right atrial dilatation. Consequently, patients with both AFMR and AFTR will require concomitant tricuspid valve repair when they undergo mitral valve repair. A valve replacement may also be a better option for the treatment of AFMR and AFTR in patients with excessive atrial dilatations. Bilateral atrioventricular valve annuloplasty alone may not be beneficial in patients who have AFMR and AFTR with apparent giant LA and RA. Atrial plication should be considered as a concomitant procedure on a patient-by-patient basis. A need for a Maze procedure should also be considered on a patient-by-patient basis. By contrast, surgery in elderly patients with AFMR and a high surgical risk is challenging. Various semi-invasive catheter device therapies may be good options for the treatment of elderly high-risk patients with AFMR.[35]

SUMMARY

AFMR can occur in atrial fibrillation patients despite a preserved LV systolic function. Our belief is that the MA dilatation owing to atrial fibrillation-induced LA dilatation is necessary for the generation of AFMR. Insufficient leaflet remodeling leads to the development of AFMR. Hamstringing of the PML also relates to the occurrence of AFMR. Further MA dilatation owing to progressive dilatations of both LA and LV with MR-induced volume overload worsens the AFMR. However, AFMR is not a homogenous disease; it can be classified into 2 types: one has the flattened AML, a flattened PML, and a central jet (Carpentier I), and the other has the flattened AML with a pseudoprolapse, a tethered PML with the hamstringing phenomenon, and an eccentric jet (Carpentier I for AML and IIIb for PML). AFMR seems to have been present in the past, but is a new disease entity that has recently become highlighted. Appropriate diagnosis and treatments need to be established.

CLINICS CARE POINTS

- Atrial functional mitral regurgitation (AFMR) can occur as a consequence of left atrial dilation in patients with atrial fibrillation.
- AFMR can be a cause of heart failure.
- AFMR can be a target of invasive therapies.

DISCLOSURE

Y. Abe, Y. Takahashi, and T. Shibata declare that they have no conflicts of interest.

REFERENCES

1. Nishimura RA, Otto CM, Bonow RO, et al. 2017 AHA/ACC focused update of the 2014 AHA/ACC Guideline for the management of patients with valvular heart disease: a report of the American College of Cardiology/American Heart Association Task Force on clinical practice guidelines. Circulation 2017; 135:e1159–95.
2. Baumgartner H, Falk V, Bax JJ, et al. 2017 ESC/EACTS Guidelines for the management of valvular heart disease. Eur Heart J 2017;38:2739–91.
3. Trichon BH, Felker GM, Shaw LK, et al. Relation of frequency and severity of mitral regurgitation to survival among patients with left ventricular systolic dysfunction and heart failure. Am J Cardiol 2003;91:538–43.
4. Robbins JD, Maniar PB, Cotts W, et al. Prevalence and severity of mitral regurgitation in chronic systolic heart failure. Am J Cardiol 2003;91:360–2.
5. Grigioni F, Enriquez-Sarano M, Zehr KJ, et al. Ischemic mitral regurgitation: long-term outcome and prognostic implications with quantitative Doppler assessment. Circulation 2001;103:1759–64.
6. Zhou X1, Otsuji Y, Yoshifuku S, et al. Impact of atrial fibrillation on tricuspid and mitral annular dilatation and valvular regurgitation. Circ J 2002;66:913–6.
7. Otsuji Y, Kumanohoso T, Yoshifuku S, et al. Isolated annular dilation does not usually cause important functional mitral regurgitation: comparison between patients with lone atrial fibrillation and those with idiopathic or ischemic cardiomyopathy. J Am Coll Cardiol 2002;39:1651–6.
8. Kihara T, Gillinov AM, Takasaki K, et al. Mitral regurgitation associated with mitral annular dilation in patients with lone atrial fibrillation: an echocardiographic study. Echocardiography 2009;26:885–9.
9. Gertz ZM, Raina A, Saghy L, et al. Evidence of atrial functional mitral regurgitation due to atrial fibrillation: reversal with arrhythmia control. J Am Coll Cardiol 2011;58:1474–81.
10. Takahashi Y, Abe Y, Sasaki Y, et al. Mitral valve repair for atrial functional mitral regurgitation in patients with chronic atrial fibrillation. Interact Cardiovasc Thorac Surg 2015;21:163–8.
11. Machino-Ohtsuka T, Seo Y, Ishizu T, et al. Novel mechanistic insights into atrial functional mitral regurgitation: 3-dimensional echocardiographic study. Circ J 2016;80:2240–8.
12. Ito K, Abe Y, Takahashi Y, et al. Mechanism of atrial functional mitral regurgitation in patients with atrial fibrillation: a study using three-dimensional transesophageal echocardiography. J Cardiol 2017;70:584–90.
13. Kagiyama N, Hayashida A, Toki M, et al. Insufficient leaflet remodeling in patients with atrial fibrillation: association with the severity of mitral regurgitation. Circ Cardiovasc Imaging 2017;10:e005451.
14. Abe Y, Akamatsu K, Ito K, et al. Prevalence and prognostic significance of functional mitral and tricuspid regurgitation despite preserved left ventricular ejection fraction in atrial fibrillation patients. Circ J 2018;82:1451–8.
15. Saito C, Minami Y, Arai K, et al. Prevalence, clinical characteristics, and outcome of atrial functional mitral regurgitation in hospitalized heart failure patients with atrial fibrillation. J Cardiol 2018;72:292–9.
16. Ito K, Abe Y, Watanabe H, et al. Prognostic significance of residual functional mitral regurgitation in hospitalized heart failure patients with chronic atrial fibrillation and preserved ejection fraction after medical therapies. J Echocardiogr 2019;17:197–205.
17. Kim DH, Heo R, Handschumacher MD, et al. Mitral valve adaptation to isolated annular dilation: insights into the mechanism of atrial functional mitral regurgitation. JACC Cardiovasc Imaging 2019;12:665–77.
18. Tang Z, Fan YT, Wang Y, et al. Mitral annular and left ventricular dynamics in atrial functional mitral regurgitation: a three-dimensional and speckle-tracking echocardiographic study. J Am Soc Echocardiogr 2019;32:503–13.
19. Silbiger JJ. Mechanistic insights into atrial functional mitral regurgitation: far more complicated than just left atrial remodeling. Echocardiography 2019;36:164–9.
20. Dziadzko V, Dziadzko M, Medina-Inojosa JR, et al. Causes and mechanisms of isolated mitral regurgitation in the community: clinical context and outcome. Eur Heart J 2019;40:2194–202.
21. Abe Y, Takahashi Y, Shibata T, et al. Functional mitral regurgitation, updated: ventricular or atrial? J Echocardiogr 2020;18:1–8.
22. Akamatsu K, Abe Y, Matsumura Y, et al. Etiology of atrial functional mitral regurgitation: insights from transthoracic echocardiography in 159 consecutive patients with atrial fibrillation and preserved left

ventricular ejection fraction. Cardiology 2020;145: 511–21.

23. Tamargo M, Obokata M, Reddy YNV, et al. Functional mitral regurgitation and left atrial myopathy in heart failure with preserved ejection fraction. Eur J Heart Fail 2020;22:489–98.

24. Kim K, Kitai T, Kaji S, et al. Outcomes and predictors of cardiac events in medically treated patients with atrial functional mitral regurgitation. Int J Cardiol 2020;316:195–202.

25. Furukawa A, Abe Y, Ito K, et al. Mechanisms of changes in functional mitral regurgitation by preload alterations. J Cardiol 2018;71:570–6.

26. Huchins GM, Moore GW, Skoog DK, et al. The association of floppy mitral valve with disjunction of the mitral annulus fibrosus. N Engl J Med 1986;314: 535–40.

27. Angelini A, Ho SY, Anderson RH, et al. A histological study of the atrioventricular junction in hearts with normal and prolapsed leaflets of the mitral valve. Br Heart J 1988;59:712–6.

28. Konda T, Tani T, Suganuma N, et al. The analysis of mitral annular disjunction detected by echocardiography and comparison with previously reported pathological data. J Echocardiogr 2017;15:176–85.

29. Chaput M, Handschumacher MD, Tournoux F, et al. Mitral leaflet adaptation to ventricular remodeling: occurrence and adequacy in patients with functional mitral regurgitation. Circulation 2008;118:845–52.

30. Dal-Bianco JP, Aikawa E, Bischoff J, et al. Active adaptation of the tethered mitral valve: insights into a compensatory mechanism for functional mitral regurgitation. Circulation 2009;120:334–42.

31. Netter FH. The CIBA collection of medical illustrations, vol. 5. Summit (NJ): CIBA; 1969. Heart.

32. Izumi C, Eishi K, Ashihara K, et al. JCS/JSCS/JATS/ JSVS 2020 guidelines on the management of valvular heart disease. Circ J 2020. https://doi.org/ 10.1253/circj.CJ-20-0135.

33. Sakaguchi T, Totsugawa T, Orihashi K, et al. Mitral annuloplasty for atrial functional mitral regurgitation in patients with chronic atrial fibrillation. J Card Surg 2019;34:767–73.

34. Takahashi Y, Abe Y, Murakami T, et al. Mid-term results of valve repairs for atrial functional mitral and tricuspid regurgitations. Gen Thorac Cardiovasc Surg 2020;68:467–76.

35. Nagaura T, Hayashi A, Yoshida J, et al. Percutaneous edge-to-edge repair for atrial functional mitral regurgitation: a real-time 3-dimensional transesophageal echocardiography study. JACC Cardiovasc Imaging 2019;12:1881–3.

Mitral Annular Disjunction—A New Disease Spectrum

Tomoko Tani, MD[a],*, Toshiko Konda, BSc[b], Takeshi Kitai, MD, PhD[c],
Mitsuhiko Ota, MD[d], Yutaka Furukawa, MD, PhD[c]

KEYWORDS

• Mitral annular disjunction • Mitral valve prolapse • Arrhythmia • Echocardiography

KEY POINTS

- Mitral annular disjunction is a structural abnormality of the mitral annulus fibrosus. It refers to a separation between the atrial wall-mitral valve junction and the left ventricular attachment defined by pathologist.
- Mitral annular disjunction is a common finding in patients with myxomatous mitral valve diseases, such as Barlow syndrome.
- Mitral annular disjunction has been recognized in relation to ventricular arrhythmia and sudden death. The width of mitral annular disjunction correlates with the incidence of nonsustained ventricular tachycardia in patients with myxomatous mitral valve diseases.
- Mitral annular disjunction itself possibly concerns to ventricular arrhythmia because of mechanical stretch. We need to perform prospective studies to reveal the meanings of mitral annular disjunction in arrhythmic mitral valve prolapse.

INTRODUCTION

Mitral annular disjunction is a structural abnormality of the mitral annulus fibrosus, which has been described by pathologists to be associated with mitral leaflet prolapse (Fig. 1).[1–3] Hutchins and colleagues,[1] in their study of 900 autopsied hearts, observed disjunction of the mitral annulus in hearts with mitral valve prolapse (MVP). They defined disjunction as a separation of the atrial wall-mitral valve (MV) junction and the attachment of the left ventricle (LV). They revealed that disjunction was an anatomic variation of the normal morphologic characteristics of the mitral annulus fibrosus, because it was present in approximately 6% of human hearts.[1] During the cardiac cycle, the region of disjunction permits the atrium-valve leaflet junction of the mitral apparatus to move outwardly in relation to the atrial aspect of the ventricular wall during ventricular systole and inwardly during ventricular diastole. Mitral annular disjunctions are also of varying degrees.

PATHOLOGY OF MITRAL ANNULAR DISJUNCTION

The histopathologic abnormality of mitral annular disjunction was first reported by Hutchins and colleagues in 1986.[1] Among 900 autopsied hearts, floppy MVs were detected in 25 hearts (2.8%). About 92% of these 25 hearts had mitral annular disjunction. In 42 other hearts (5%) from significantly younger patients, there were mitral annular disjunctions without floppy MVs. They defined

[a] Basic Medical Science, Kobe City College of Nursing, 3-4 Gakuennishi-machi, Nishi-ku, Kobe 651-2103, Japan; [b] Department of Clinical Technology, Kobe City Medical Center General Hospital, 2-1-1 Minatojima-Minamimachi, Chuo-ku, Kobe 650-0047, Japan; [c] Department of Cardiovaasucular Medicine, Kobe City Medical Center General Hospital, 2-1-1 Minatojima-Minamimachi, Chuo-ku, Kobe 650-0047, Japan; [d] Department of Cardiovascular Center, Toranomon Hospital, 2-2-2 Toranomon, Minato-ku, Tokyo 105-8470, Japan
* Corresponding author.
E-mail address: tomokot@tr.kobe-ccn.ac.jp

Cardiol Clin 39 (2021) 289–294
https://doi.org/10.1016/j.ccl.2021.01.011
0733-8651/21/© 2021 Elsevier Inc. All rights reserved.

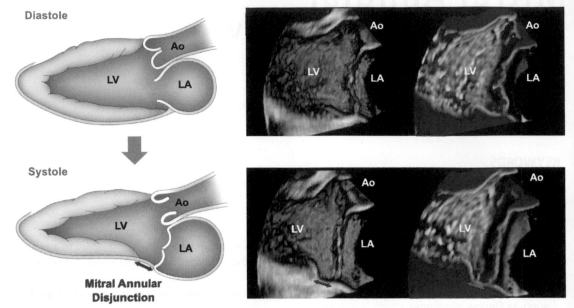

Fig. 1. Mitral annular disjunction (*arrow*). Measurement of mitral annular disjunction is recommended to be performed at end-systolic phase. Ao, aorta; LA, left atrium; LV, left ventricle.

mitral annular disjunction as a separation of the atrial wall-MV junction and the LV attachment.[1] In 1988, Angelini and Becker reported that there was no significant difference in the number of segments around the left atrioventricular junction, which showed disjunction in hearts with normal or prolapsing leaflets.[2] They also pointed out that mitral annular disjunction is an anatomic variation of the normal morphologic characteristics of the mitral annulus, seen in floppy valves, as reported by Hutchins.[2] In addition, they suggested that if hypermobility of the mitral apparatus is important in producing prolapse, it is probably produced by other abnormalities over and above so-called disjunction.[2]

ANATOMY AND PHYSIOLOGY OF THE MITRAL ANNULUS AND MITRAL ANNULAR DISJUNCTION

The aortic valve continues fibrously with the anterior leaflet of the MV and the right and left fibrous trigones. This region of the annulus is fibrous and less prone to dilatation. The remaining two-thirds of the annulus is composed of muscle and dilate easily in patients with mitral regurgitation (MR). Therefore, we can detect mitral annular displacement mainly in the posterior leaflet. This part of the mitral annulus may represent an area weakened by mechanical stress.

Normally, the posterior mitral ring and its adjacent myocardium moves synchronously with the LV. On the contrary, when the mitral annulus is

disjunctive, annuloventricular coupling is not preserved and the mitral annulus moves abnormally. Left ventricular wall curling has been defined as an unusual systolic motion of the posterior mitral ring on the adjacent myocardium.[4]

The quantitative assessment of curling by cardiac magnetic resonance imaging (CMR) was defined as a perpendicular distance from a line between the top of LV inferobasal wall and the LA wall-posterior MV leaflet junction to the lower limit of the mitral annulus during end-systole. Perazzolo Marra and colleagues reported that curling of the mitral annulus is associated with mitral annular disjunction. There was a linear correlation between the length of mitral annular disjunction and the severity of curling.[4]

DIAGNOSIS OF MITRAL ANNULAR DISJUNCTION

Usually, we can detect mitral annular disjunction on parasternal long-axis view by transthoracic echocardiography. During the cardiac cycle, this region of disjunction permits the atrium-valve leaflet junction of the mitral apparatus to move outwardly in relation to the atrial aspect of the ventricular wall during ventricular systole and inwardly during ventricular diastole. The mitral annular disjunction distance was usually measured during the end-systolic phase in the parasternal long-axis view. We previously reported 2.0 mm as the minimum value of mitral annular disjunction by which measurement is possible.[5] When multiple sonographers measured the same cases with mitral annular disjunction, all sonographers could recognize the presence of mitral annular disjunction and could measure the distance when it was greater than 2 mm.[5] Lee and colleagues[6] reported that mitral annular disjunction was located adjacent to the prolapsed segments, circumferentially spanning over average 87° of the annulus on 3-dimensional (3D) transesophageal echocardiography.

CMR is also useful in detecting mitral annular disjunction. Mitral annular disjunction can be detected on the apical 4 chamber in midventricular systole. Dejgaard and colleagues[7] reported that a complete assessment of the mitral annulus circumference can be made by using 6 LV long-axis cine sequences with an interslice rotation of 30°. In that study, the longitudinal mitral annular disjunction distance was 3.0 mm and the circumferential mitral annular disjunction was 150°. They showed that mitral annular disjunction could be detected in up to two-thirds of the mitral ring circumference.[7] An advantage of CMR is that it can be used to evaluate arrhythmogenic left ventricular walls with the aid of late gadolinium enhancement (LGE) in contrast-enhanced CMR (CE-CMR). They also identified the presence of basolateral left ventricular wall curling motion by visual assessment in parasternal long-axis view, apical long-axis view, and apical 4-chamber view by echocardiography.[7] Recently, Putnam and colleagues[8] reported that cardiac computed tomography (CCT) can be used to detect mitral annular disjunction. In that study, a 256-slice multidetector CT scanner was used and then multiplanar reconstruction (MPR) was performed. Using MPR, they could determine the presence and measure the distance of mitral annular disjunction. Future research of CT is expected.[8]

MITRAL VALVE PROLAPSE AND MITRAL ANNULAR DISJUNCTION

We previously reported that mitral annular disjunction was detected not only in patients with a myxomatous MV but also in normal cases, and the frequency of MVP was significantly larger in patients with mitral annular disjunction than in those without it. Mitral annular disjunction was detected in 28% of patients with MVP.[5]

There were 8 reports that investigated the prevalence and clinical outcomes among patients with mitral annular disjunction (**Table 1**). Firstly, Eriksson and colleagues performed a retrospective analysis of the intraoperative transesophageal echocardiography in 67 patients with advanced mitral valvular degeneration. They also analyzed a subgroup of 32 patients with mild/moderate mitral valvular degeneration.[9] They reported that

mitral annular disjunction was detected at the base of the posterior leaflet in 98% of patients with advanced and in 9% of patients with mild/moderate mitral valvular degeneration.[9] Lee and colleagues studied 101 patients with MVP, 30 subjects with normal MV, and 25 heart failure patients with functional MR using real-time 3D transesophageal echocardiography and detected mitral annular disjunction in 42 patients with mVP (42%).[6] They also evaluated mitral annular motion and observed that when the annulus was disjunctive, its motion no longer followed LV contraction, but it exhibited paradoxic dynamics, conforming to atrial wall motion. They concluded that the disjunctive annulus was decoupled functionally from the ventricle, leading to paradoxic annular dynamics with systolic expansion and flattening, that may require specific intervention.[6] Recently, Putnam and colleagues studied 90 patients with MVP and severe MR, who had preoperative CCT.[8] The presence of mitral annular disjunction was associated with female gender, smaller annulus size, and greater posterior leaflet length.[8] Mategazza and colleagues concluded that mitral annular disjunction could be detected in a minority of patients with fibroelastic deficiency and not only patients with Barlow disease. The feasibility of MV repair was no different between these groups.[10]

ARRHYTHMIC MITRAL VALVE PROLAPSE AND MITRAL ANNULAR DISJUNCTION

Basso and colleagues[11] reported the autopsy findings of 43 sudden cardiac death patients with isolated MVP and observed bileaflet involvement in 70% of them. Fibrosis of the papillary muscles and inferobasal LV wall correlates with the origins of ventricular arrhythmias.[11] Arrhythmic MVP should be clearly distinguished from echocardiographic MVP. There are various opinions of mechanism. Excessive mobility of leaflets causes mechanical stretching of the mitral annulus.[12] It concerns left ventricular fibrosis.[13] Miller reported that bileaflet MVP is a high-risk feature for sudden cardiac death. Mitral annular disjunction was considered to be a constant feature of arrhythmic MVP with LV fibrosis.[14] Parazzollo Marra and colleagues reported that mitral annular disjunction was significantly longer in MVP patients with LGE on CE-CMR than in those without it. Longer mitral annular disjunction was detected in 50 sudden death patients with MVP and fibrosis than in 20 patients without MVP. Mitral annular disjunction was detected in both patients with arrhythmic MVP with LV LGE and sudden cardiac death cases with LV fibrosis. Mitral annular disjunction and curling were confirmed by histology in sudden cardiac

Table 1
Prevalence of mitral annular disjunction in some studies

First Author	Study Design	Year	Imaging	Diagnosis	Characteristics of Population	Rate of Mitral Annular Disjunction
Erikisson et al,[9] 2005	Retrospective cohort study	1991–1995	TEE	Myxomatous mitral valve disease	n: 67 Mean age: 52 y Female 34%	Advanced MVD: 31/32 (97%) Mild/moderate MVD: 3/32 (9%)
Carmo et al,[15] 2010	Retrospective cohort study	2003–2006	TTE	Myxomatous mitral valve disease	n: 38 Mean age: 57 y Female 47%	21/38 (55%)
Perazzolo Marra et al,[4] 2016	Retrospective cohort study	2010–2014	CE-CMR	MVP	n: 52 Mean age: 44 y Female 63%	37/52 (71%)
Lee et al,[6] 2017	Retrospective cohort study		TEE	MVP, FMR, and normal control	n: 156 Mean age: 58 y Female 33%	42/156 (27%)
Konda et al,[5] 2017	Retrospective cohort study	2014	TTE	Refferred TTE	n: 1439 Mean age: 65 y Female 42%	125/1439 (9%)
Dejgaard et al,[7] 2018	Cross-sectional study	2015–2017	TTE and CE-CMR	Patients with mitral annular disjunction	n:116 Mean age: 49 y Female 70%	
Mantegazza et al,[10] 2019			TTE	MVP and severe MR	n: 979 Mean age: 63 y	103/979 (16.2%)
Putnam et al,[8] 2020	Retrospective cohort study	2013–2019	Cardiac CT	MVP and severe MR	n: 90 Mean age: 63 y Female 26%	18/90 (20%)
Konda et al,[17] 2020	Retrospective cohort study	2009–2010	TTE	MVP and severe MR	n: 185 Mean age: 62 y Female 40%	45/185 (24%)

Abbreviations: CE-CMR, contrast-enhanced cardiac magnetic resonance; FMR, functional mitral regurgitation; MVD, mitral valve disease; MVP, mitral valve prolapse; TEE, transesophageal echocardiography; TTE, transthoracic echocardiography.

death patients with MVP. Excessive mobility of the leaflets and systolic curling have clinical important implications. They concluded that mitral annular disjunction is associated with arrhythmic MVP.[4] Carmo and colleagues[15] found that the severity of mitral annular disjunction significantly correlated with the occurrence of nonsustained ventricular tachycardia (NSVT), and a disjunction of greater than 8.5 mm was predictive of NSVT. Essayagh and colleagues showed that ventricular arrhythmia were frequent in patients with MVP but rarely severe in those with only MR. They concluded that arrhythmic MVP was strongly associated with specific electrocardiographic (ECG) changes, the presence of mitral annular disjunction, and leaflet redundancy but was independent of MR severity.[16] Dejgaard and colleagues investigated CMR and 24-hour ECG recordings in patients with mitral annular disjunction. About 54% of patients with mitral annular disjunction had MVP. There was no difference in the prevalence of ventricular arrhythmias between those mitral disjunction patients with MVP and those without MVP. They reported that the longitudinal distance of mitral annular disjunction in the posterolateral wall and papillary muscle fibrosis assessed by CMR were predictive of ventricular arrhythmia. They concluded that mitral annular disjunction itself was an arrhythmogenic entity.[7] According to previous studies, the site of mitral annular disjunction may become the origin of arrhythmias. We studied 185 patients with severe MR caused by fibroelastic deficiency and Barlow syndrome. Mitral annular disjunction was detected in 24% patients with severe MR. During a median follow-up of 20.3 years, arrhythmic events and sudden death occurred in 7 patients (3.8%). The number of patients with cardiac events were significantly larger in the group that received medical treatment ($P = .02$). All patients had no mitral annular disjunction. In this study, we investigated for the patients with severe MR limitedly. Therefore, we need to investigate for patients with various MR grade to clarify the significance of mitral annular disjunction.[17]

CLINICAL IMPLICATIONS

The presence of mitral annular disjunction means with hypermobility of the mitral apparatus. Loose connection between the junction of the MV and the LV results in hypermobility of the posterior mitral annulus and may be associated with MVP. Flameng and colleagues[18] reported the importance of using sliding plasty in MV surgery for posterior displacement of the mitral annulus. Newcomb and colleagues concluded that correction of the annular dilation and posterior displacement, shortening of

the height of the posterior leaflet, and correction of valvular prolapse provided excellent functional results. They reported that advanced myxomatous degeneration is an independent predictor of repair failure due to inadequate annuloplasty. Posterior annular displacement, which means mitral annular disjunction, may be another cause of repair failure[19] Fixation of the hyperenhanced annular dynamics using ring annuloplasty may be sufficient to restore MV competence.

Mitral annular disjunction has been reported to be associated with ventricular arrhythmia and sudden cardiac death. If mitral annular disjunction is incidentally detected in patients during echocardiography, we have to evaluate for features and a history of arrhythmia. If necessary, a Holter ECG should be performed. The presence and importance of mitral annular disjunction should be spread. The clinical and physiologic meanings of mitral annular disjunction and MVP is an important work in progress. The molecular mechanism should be investigated.[20]

SUMMARY

Mitral annular disjunction is a structural abnormality that is seen not only in patients with myxomatous MVs but also is in patients with MVP. The prevalence of mitral annular disjunction should be checked routinely during presurgical imaging. Otherwise, mitral annular disjunction itself might be an arrhythmogenic entity, irrespective of the presence of MVP. Therefore, we should check echocardiography keeping in mind mitral annular disjunction. Further prospective studies are needed to address whether a causative mechanistic link exists between mitral annular disjunction and arrhythmic MVP or severe MR.

CLINICS CARE POINTS

- Check the presence of mitral annular disjunction in every patient particularly with mitral valve disease because mitral annular disjunction itself is arrhythmogenic.

DISCLOSURE

All authors have nothing to disclose.

REFERENCES

1. Hutchins GM, Moore GW, Skoog DK. The association of floppy mitral valve with disjunction of the mitral annulus fibrosus. N Engl J Med 1986;314:535–40.

2. Angelini A, Ho SY, Anderson RH, et al. A histological study of the atrioventricular junction in hearts with normal and prolapsed leaflets of the mitral valve. Br Heart J 1988;59:712–6.

3. Becker AE, De Wit AP. Mitral valve apparatus. A spectrum of normality relevant to mitral valve prolapse. Br Heart J 1979;42:680–9.

4. Perazzolo Marra M, Basso C, De Lazzari M, et al. Morphofunctional abnormalities of mitral annulus and arrhythmic mitral valve prolapse. Cir Cardiovasc Imaging 2016;9:e005030.

5. Konda T, Tani T, Suganuma N, et al. The analysis of mitral annular disjunction detected by echocardiography and comparison with previously reported pathological data. J Echocardiogr 2017;15:176–85.

6. Lee AP, Jin CN, Fan Y, et al. Functional implication of mitral annular disjunction in mitral valve prolapse: a quantitative dynamic 3D echocardiographic study. JACC Cardiovasc Imaging 2017;10:1424–33.

7. Dejgaard LA, Skjølsvik ET, Lie ØH, et al. The mitral annulus disjunction arrhythmic syndrome. J Am Coll Cardiol 2018;72:1600–9.

8. Putnam AJ, Kebed K, Mor-Avi V, et al. Prevalence of mitral annular disjunction in patients with mitral valve prolapse and severe regurgitation. Int J Cardiovasc Imaging 2020;36:1363–70.

9. Eriksson MJ, Bitkover CY, Omran AS, et al. Mitral annular disjunction in advanced myxomatous mitral valve disease: echocardiographic detection and surgical correction. J Am Soc Echocardiogr 2005; 18:1014–22.

10. Mantegazza V, Tamborini G, Muratori M, et al. Mitral annular disjunction in a large cohort of patients with mitral valve prolapse and significant regurgitation. JACC Cardiovasc Imaging 2019;12:2278–80.

11. Basso C, Perazzolo Marra M, Rizzo S, et al. Arrhythmic mitral valve prolapse and sudden cardiac death. Circulation 2015;132:556–66.

12. Han HC, Ha FJ, Teh AW, et al. Mitral valve prolapse and sudden cardiac death. A systematic review. J Am Heart Assoc 2018;7:e010584.

13. Nalliah CJ, Mahajan R, Elliott AD, et al. Mitral valve prolapse and sudden cardiac death: a systematic review and meta-analysis. Heart 2018;105:144–51.

14. Miller MA, Dukkipati SR, Turagam M, et al. Arrhythmic mitral valve prolapse: JACC review topic of the week. J Am Coll Cardiol 2018;72:2904–14.

15. Carmo P, Andrade MJ, Aguiar C, et al. Mitral annular disjunction in myxomatous mitral valve disease: a relevant abnormality recognizable by transthoracic echocardiography. Cardiovasc Ultrasound 2010;8:53.

16. Essayagh B, Sabbag A, Antoine C, et al. Presentation and outcome of arrhythmic mitral valve prolapse. J Am Coll Cardiol 2020;76:637–49.

17. Konda T, Tani T, Suganuma N, et al. Mitral annular disjunction in patients with primary severe mitral regurgitation and mitral valve prolapse. Echocardiography 2020;37(11):1716–22.

18. Flameng W, Meuris B, Herijers P, et al. Durability of mitral valve repair in Barlow disease versus fibroelastic deficiency. J Thorac Cardiovasc Surg 2008; 135:274–82.

19. Newcomb AE, David TE, Lad VS, et al. Mitral valve repair for advanced myxomatous degeneration with posterior displacement of the mitral annulus. J Thorac Cardiovasc Surg 2008;136:1503–9.

20. Enriquez-Sarano M. Mitral annular disjunction: the forgotten component of myxomatous mitral valve disease. JACC Cardiovasc Imaging 2017;10: 1434–6.

Moving?

Make sure your subscription moves with you!

To notify us of your new address, find your **Clinics Account Number** (located on your mailing label above your name), and contact customer service at:

Email: journalscustomerservice-usa@elsevier.com

800-654-2452 (subscribers in the U.S. & Canada)
314-447-8871 (subscribers outside of the U.S. & Canada)

Fax number: 314-447-8029

Elsevier Health Sciences Division
Subscription Customer Service
3251 Riverport Lane
Maryland Heights, MO 63043

*To ensure uninterrupted delivery of your subscription, please notify us at least 4 weeks in advance of move.

Printed and bound by CPI Group (UK) Ltd, Croydon, CR0 4YY

03/10/2024

01040308-0013